VET UPDATE

CONGESTIVE HEART FAILURE

edra

Copyright © 2019 Grupo Asís Biomedia, SL
Plaza Antonio Beltrán Martínez nº 1, planta 8 - letra I
(Centro empresarial El Trovador)
50002 Zaragoza - Spain

First printing: January 2019

This book was originally published in Spanish under the title:
Servet update. Insuficiencia cardiaca congestiva
© 2018 Grupo Asís Biomedia, SL
ISBN Spanish edition: 978-84-17225-40-7

Translation:
Lori Newman

Illustrator:
Jacob Gragera Artal

ISBN: 978-84-17225-75-9
DL: Z 1092-2018

Design, layout and printing:
Grupo Asís Biomedia, SL
www.grupoasis.com
info@grupoasis.com

GRUPO asis

Warning:

Veterinary science is constantly evolving, as are pharmacology and the other sciences. Inevitably, it is therefore the responsibility of the veterinary surgeon to determine and verify the dosage, the method of administration, the duration of treatment and any possible contraindications to the treatments given to each individual patient, based on his or her professional experience. Neither the publisher nor the author can be held liable for any damage or harm caused to people, animals or properties resulting from the correct or incorrect application of the information contained in this book.

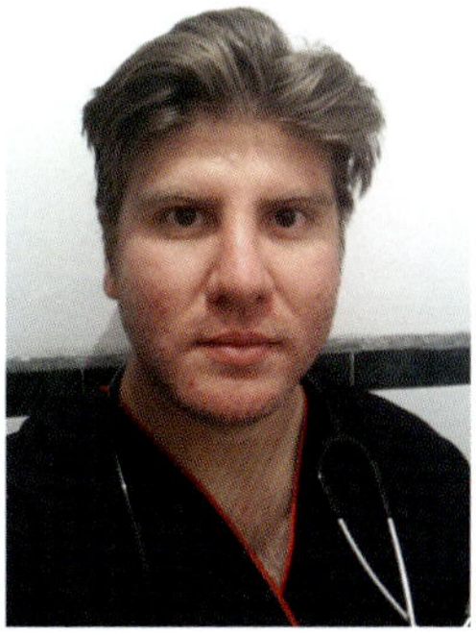

THE AUTHOR

Javier Esteban Rodríguez Velarde

Javier Esteban Rodríguez Velarde earned his degree in veterinary medicine from the Universidad Agraria of Ecuador in 2006. He trained in the Cardiology Service at the California Animal Hospital (United States) and in other cardiology and ultrasound services in both human and veterinary medicine. He was a veterinary clinician at Lucky veterinary hospital, Quito (Ecuador), from 2006 to 2010, where he founded the cardiology and ultrasound service and served as medical director from 2010 until 2015. Since 2011, he has been a professor at the Faculty of Veterinary Medicine of the Universidad San Francisco (USFQ) of Quito and a cardiologist and ultrasonographer at the USFQ Veterinary Specialty Hospital. He is currently medical director of the Cardiomedicc veterinary cardiology and ultrasound centre. He has lectured on cardiology, ultrasonography, and intensive care in more than 40 courses and international conferences in Ecuador and elsewhere.

PREFACE

Cardiomyopathies are common in dogs. Approximately 10 % of dogs seen in veterinary practice in North America present with cardiac disease. Among these patients, some will develop congestive heart failure (CHF), and a subset of those will require hospitalisation for acute decompensation.

Congestive heart failure is a clinical syndrome characterised by clinical signs related to fluid retention and/or low cardiac output resulting from structural or functional diseases of the heart.

The principal clinical signs are tachypnoea, dyspnoea, cough, abdominal distension due to ascites, hindlimb oedema, exercise intolerance, weakness, fatigue, and syncope. These are common presenting complaints in small animal practice. Causes of CHF in dogs may be both congenital and acquired; they include valvular, myocardial, and pericardial diseases, as well as vascular diseases and left-right shunts.

Progress in understanding and treating CHF in dogs has enhanced the quality of life and expected survival of affected individuals. As a result of these advances, a systematic review of the different aspects of this syndrome is necessary.

The goal of this guide is to provide small animal cardiologists as well as internal medicine and emergency and critical care specialists with current information on the pathophysiology and clinical manifestations of CHF, together with important resources for diagnosis and recommendations for treating dogs with this disease.

I hope this guide will improve understanding of this syndrome and support timely decision-making during diagnosis and treatment.

Given the difficulty of including all relevant scientific material in this guide and the inability to address every aspect of the topic in one volume, I invite the reader to review the remaining literature (both articles and books) that I was unable to include here.

The unceasing flow of scientific publications and advances in the field of veterinary cardiology mean we must remain abreast of updates following the publication of this guide.

Javier Esteban Rodríguez Velarde

TABLE OF CONTENTS

DEFINITION

One of the most significant cardiology associations in the world, the American College of Cardiology/American Heart Association, defines congestive heart failure (CHF) as a complex clinical syndrome that arises from any structural or functional cardiac disease that impedes the ventricle's ability to fill with or eject blood. The principal manifestations of CHF are dyspnoea and fatigue, which can induce exercise intolerance and promote fluid retention, resulting in pulmonary congestion and peripheral oedema. While both pulmonary congestion and peripheral oedema can hamper a patient's function and quality of life, they may not coincide clinically. Some patients present with exercise intolerance and minimal fluid retention, while others initially present with oedema and develop dyspnoea and fatigue only later.

CHF is a clinical syndrome characterised by fluid retention and/or low cardiac output resulting from structural or functional diseases of the heart. The severity of cardiac alterations induces an increase in the chamber filling pressures, leading to venous congestion and the resulting clinical signs, as well as a decrease in the ventricular ejection fraction and in oxygen delivery to the tissues.

PATHOPHYSIOLOGY

Knowledge of the pathophysiology of CHF will enable clinicians to understand the mechanisms by which patients develop clinical signs of CHF and how these can be treated.

CHF is a clinical syndrome with systemic manifestations and effects on multiple organs and body systems. This syndrome stems from structural or functional alterations to the heart. The main diseases that can cause these cardiac alterations in dogs are as follows:

- Congenital diseases: patent ductus arteriosus, ventricular septal defect (VSD), tricuspid valve dysplasia, subaortic stenosis, and pulmonary stenosis.
- Acquired diseases: myxomatous degeneration of the mitral valve (MV), dilated cardiomyopathy (DCM), bacterial endocarditis, and pulmonary arterial hypertension, among others. Arrhythmias such as atrial fibrillation may be secondary to structural disease (e.g. mitral insufficiency), but they can profoundly alter cardiac function and worsen the patient's clinical condition.

MECHANISMS

To illustrate the mechanisms involved in CHF, myxomatous MV degeneration and DCM will be provided as examples of structural and functional alterations, respectively.

Let us first consider the onset of MV regurgitation. Under normal conditions, during systole, the left ventricle (LV) ejects blood though the aortic valve (AV) into the systemic circulation. When MV regurgitation occurs, only a fraction of the blood ejected by the LV passes through the AV, and the rest returns to the left atrium (LA) by flowing through the regurgitant area formed by the edges of the AV leaflets. As a result, the ejection fraction and the cardiac output decrease. As valve damage progresses, the regurgitant volume increases.

In the second example, DCM functionally diminishes ventricular myocadial contractility, resulting in a decreased blood volume ejected into the systemic circulation and a decline in cardiac output.

CHF tends to evoke thoughts of significantly altered myocardial contractility, yet many patients actually have relatively normal ventricular systolic function. Ventricular diastolic function, in contrast, is always altered in CHF patients.

COMPENSATORY MECHANISMS

Decreased cardiac output occurs in both cases even though they result from rather distinct cardiac alterations. Regardless of the cause, the animal's body recognises this drop in cardiac output and activates compensatory, or adaptive, mechanisms that are ultimately detrimental to overall cardiac function. These compensatory mechanisms include neurohumoral activation (sympathetic nervous system and renin–angiotensin–aldosterone system [RAAS] activation) and cardiac remodelling; these aim to maintain normal arterial blood pressure and improve or preserve cardiac output (Fig. 1).

Neurohumoral activation

The increase in sympathetic tone begins with the fall in cardiac output, which ultimately produces clinical CHF. An increase in catecholamine concentration initially causes peripheral vasoconstriction to maintain tissue perfusion and an increase in heart rate and contractility to enhance cardiac output (positive chronotropic and inotropic effects). These effects initially compensate for the patient's clinical condition but eventually result in deterioration of cardiac function.

Arteriolar vasoconstriction causes a sustained increase in afterload, which in turn elevates systolic wall stress, resulting in myocardial hypertrophy and generalised LV systolic dysfunction (Laplace's law [Fig. 2]). Prolonged systemic vasoconstriction elevates the LV systolic pressure, resulting in myocardial hypertrophy to offset this wall stress.

$$T\ wall = \frac{P \times r}{2 \times h}$$

T wall = systolic wall stress; P = ventricular pressure; r = ventricular radius; h = wall thickness.

Figure 2. Laplace's law.

Venous vasoconstriction increases venous return and filling of the cardiac chambers (preload), which in turn increases contractility and cardiac output according to the Frank–Starling law. This progressive increase can also elevate venous and capillary pressures, resulting in clinical signs of congestion.

The increase in heart rate and contractility increases myocardial oxygen consumption while decreasing the diastolic time and, thus, the ventricular myocardial perfusion time (inducing coronary hypoperfusion). At the same

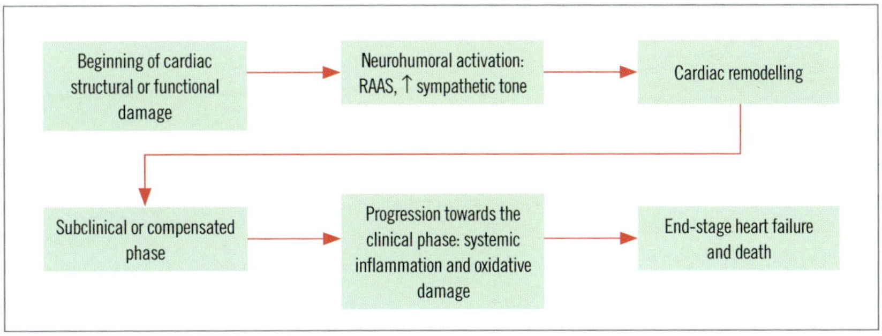

Figure 1. CHF pathophysiology.

time, the increase in the myocardial mass raises the demand for coronary blood flow. The increased myocardial oxygen demand and decreased oxygen delivery induce an ischaemia that fosters arrhythmias and myocardial fatigue. The abnormal automaticity and re-entry phenomena (resulting from heightened sympathetic tone) also favour arrhythmias.

In addition to the ischaemic phenomena, chronic myocardial exposure to high levels of catecholamines (produced by increased sympathetic tone) causes internalisation or down-regulation of B1 receptors, as well as a surfeit of G-inhibitory protein, which both minimise the effects of agonists on the B1 receptor. The result is a negative inotropic effect and an insufficient contractile response in the face of increasing catecholamine concentrations.

Along with these trends, concentrations of antidiuretic hormone and endothelin rise and RAAS activation occurs, maximising vasoconstriction and stimulating sodium and water retention.

Renin–angiotensin–aldosterone system

The RAAS is one of the pillars of neurohumoral activation. Decreased blood flow to the afferent renal artery (due to lower cardiac output), as well as sympathetic activation and hyponatraemia, stimulate renal production of renin (Fig. 3).

Renin converts angiotensinogen (an acute phase reactive protein produced in the liver) to angiotensin I, which is transformed into angiotensin II by the angiotensin-converting enzyme. Angiotensin II induces greater biological effects, namely:

- Increased sympathetic tone.
- Potent vasoconstriction and vascular remodelling (hypertrophy of the tunica media).
- Ventricular remodelling.
- Increased aldosterone production in the adrenal cortex.

These vascular phenomena increase afterload and wall stress, leading to ventricular dysfunction and increased risk of ischaemia and arrhythmia.

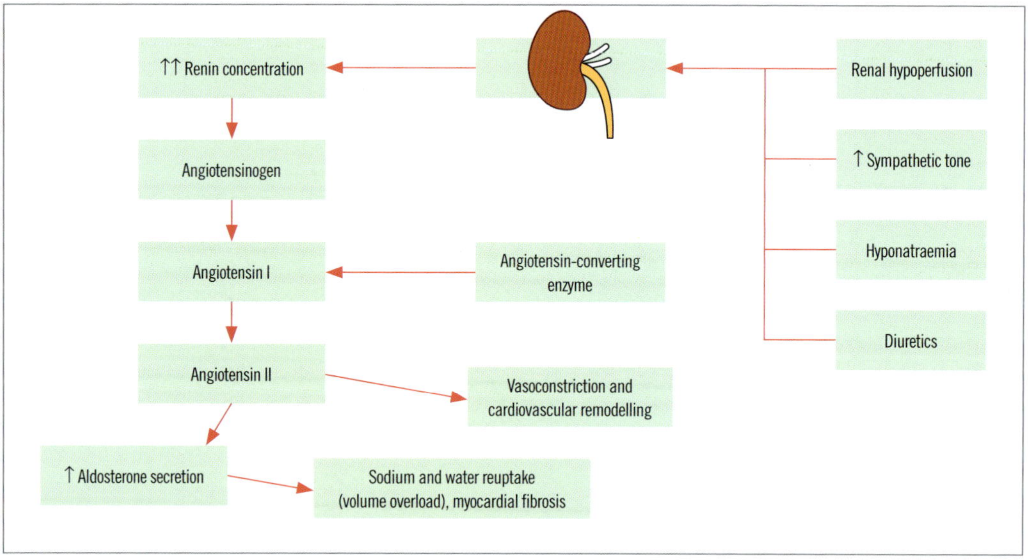

Figure 3. Renin–angiotensin–aldosterone system activation and its effects.

Aldosterone is synthesised in the adrenal cortex under the stimulation of angiotensin II or increased serum potassium. Aldosterone induces sodium reabsorption and potassium excretion in the distal renal tubule, resulting in an increased plasma volume. Aldosterone additionally enhances the catecholamine response, decreases baroreceptor sensitivity, promotes systemic inflammation, and induces myocardial and vascular fibrosis (due to its effects on cardiovascular remodelling). Treatment of CHF includes angiotensin-converting enzyme inhibiting drugs that decrease angiotensin II and aldosterone production for a certain period, since aldosterone levels will again rise despite treatment. This is referred to as aldosterone escape and has significant therapeutic implications.

Other substances involved in neurohumoral activation

Antidiuretic hormone (ADH, arginine vasopressin) is also involved in the pathophysiology of CHF. Sympathetic activation and RAAS activation stimulate ADH release from the posterior pituitary (nonosmotic stimuli). Antidiuretic hormone induces retention of free water in the renal collecting ducts, expanding the plasma volume while also producing vasoconstriction.

The intense neurohumoral activation associated with pressure or volume overload is additionally fuelled by the release of **natriuretic peptides**, which have vasodilatory, diuretic, and lusitropic (favouring diastolic function) effects to counteract overload. Atrial natriuretic peptide and B natriuretic peptide are discussed here. Atrial natriuretic peptide release from the cardiomyocyte increases as stress on the atrial wall (mainly due to atrial dilation) increases, whereas BNP release increases with elevated stress on the atrial and ventricular walls. As neurohumoral activation and tension on the cardiomyocyte increase, natriuretic peptide release increases, such that the amount of natriuretic peptide released correlates with the severity of CHF.

> Despite the beneficial effects of natriuretic peptides, they do not mitigate the deleterious effects of neurohumoral mechanisms, and CHF progresses.

Inflammatory processes, oxidative stress, and apoptosis are all now recognised as profoundly influencing progression to CHF with clinical signs. Although these factors may be present from disease onset or may result from extracardiac disease, they are amplified in the late stages of CHF. Features of late-stage CHF, such as increased wall stress, myocardial hypoxia and ischaemia, strongly stimulate the synthesis of **cytokines** such as interleukins and tumour necrosis factor. Inflammatory activation has many effects, such as mitochondrial and endothelial dysfunction, decreased capacity for calcium reuptake by the sarcoplasmic reticulum, oxidative phenomena, and programmed cell death. The result is progressive ventricular systolic and diastolic dysfunction, as well as a catabolic state called cardiac cachexia that is characterised by significant loss of muscle mass.

Cardiac remodelling and congestion

Ventricular remodelling involves dilation of the chamber and an increase in myocardial mass. This results in a higher end-diastolic volume and improved contractility (due to Starling's law), allowing the heart to eject a greater volume during systole.

Dilation of the cardiac chambers is mainly a result of increased venous return caused by a higher plasma volume. The ventricle initially adapts to this volume with no increase in the end-diastolic pressure, but the continued increase in blood volume causes this pressure to exceed physiological levels and ultimately induces ventricular hypertrophy and rigidity (products of myocardial fibrosis). The MV is open during diastole, and the mitral annulus presents minimal resistance to diastolic flow. However, ventricular pressure is transmitted to the atrium and pulmonary veins and capillaries. As the most permeable structure involved in the system, pulmonary capillaries filter fluid from the vascular space to the lung parenchyma (to the interstitial space and then the alveoli). The lymphatic system initially increases drainage of this excess fluid. However, when hydrostatic pressure in the pulmonary capillaries becomes very high, this compensatory mechanism is overwhelmed, and excess pulmonary extravascular fluid accumulates (pulmonary oedema). Left ventricular end-diastolic pressures above 25 mmHg promote fluid leakage from the vascular space to the lung parenchyma (Fig. 4). This condition is known as left-sided CHF.

In structural pathologies that alter the right side of the heart, the mechanisms of neurohumoral activation and remodelling closely resemble those described above. Increased right ventricular end-diastolic volumes induce congestion/systemic venous hypertension (in the venae cavae, hepatic veins, etc.), leading to hepatomegaly, ascites, and pleural effusion. Right ventricular end-diastolic pressures above 15 mmHg promote fluid leakage from systemic capillaries into the interstices of organs such as the liver, as well as abdominal and thoracic cavities (Fig. 5). This condition is known as right-sided CHF.

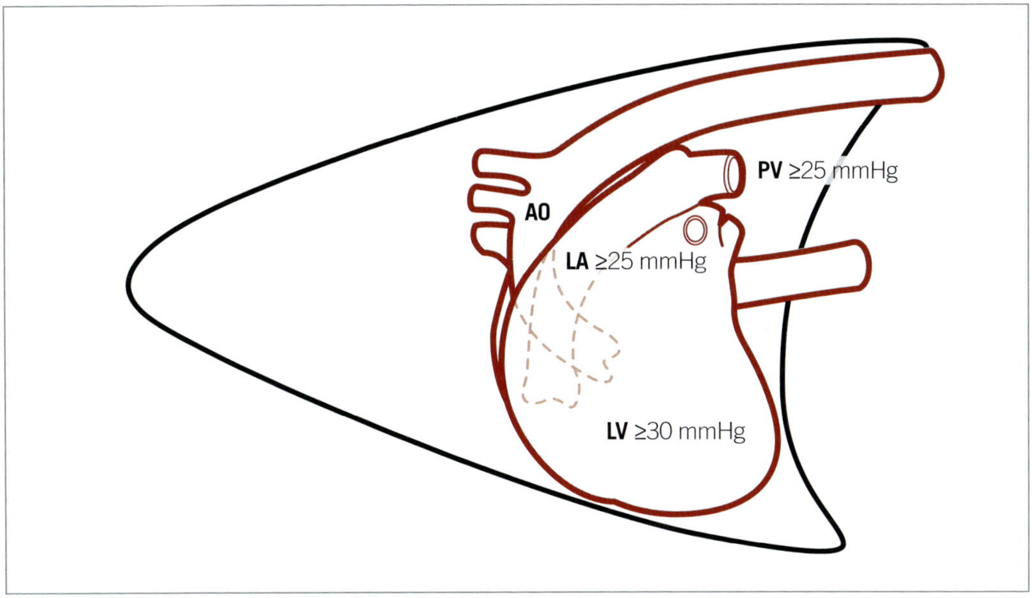

Figure 4. Left-sided congestive heart failure. Left ventricular (LV) end-diastolic pressure, mean left atrial (LA) pressure, and pulmonary venous pressure are all elevated. PV, pulmonary vein; AO, aorta.

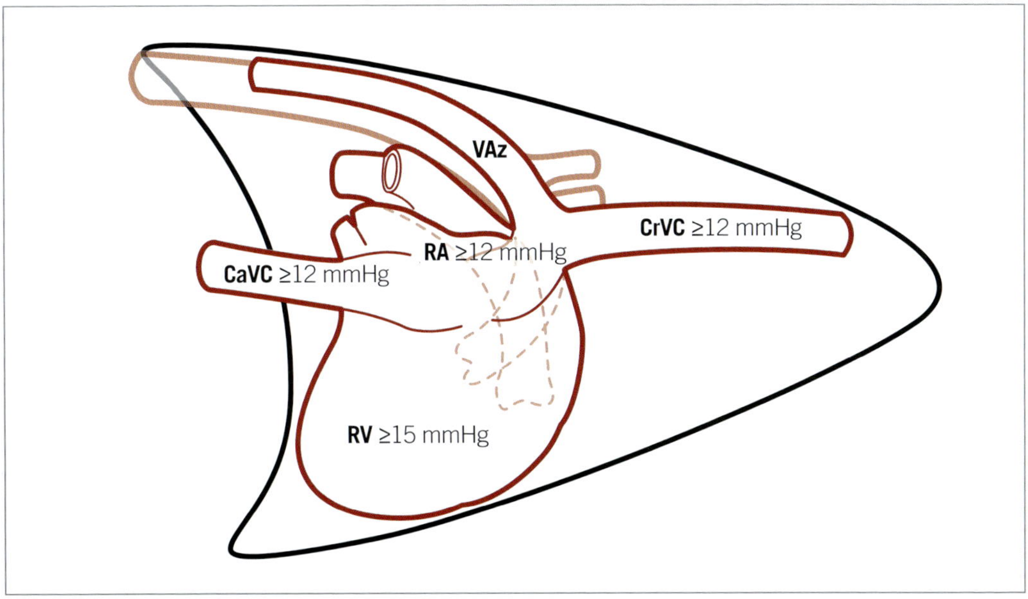

Figure 5. Right-sided congestive heart failure. Right ventricular (RV) end-diastolic pressure, mean right atrial (RA) pressure, and systemic venous pressure are all elevated. CaVC, caudal vena cava; CrVC, cranial vena cava; VAz, azygos vein.

CLINICAL APPROACH

EVALUATION OF CLINICAL SIGNS

The main presenting complaints in dogs that may be related to CHF are summarised in Table 1.

Respiratory clinical signs

Dyspnoea, tachypnoea, and cough may appear in dogs with both CHF and primary respiratory diseases, often complicating diagnosis. The physical examination may reveal signs that link the respiratory insufficiency to cardiac disease (e.g. detection of a murmur). However, some CHF patients lack a murmur, and some patients with murmurs do not have CHF. A patient may have both severe respiratory disease (of the lung parenchyma or pleural cavity) and mild cardiac disease. In this situation, the clinical signs result from the respiratory disease rather than the cardiac disease.

A murmur is not a differentiating or conclusive sign for diagnosis.

Thus, a presumptive diagnosis of CHF requires objective evaluation of cardiac structure and function, as well as of the effects of heart failure.

Respiratory signs in dogs with CHF mainly stem from pulmonary oedema or pleural effusion; however, patients with severe ascites may also present with tachypnoea and dyspnoea due to their tense abdomen restricting diaphragmatic contraction.

Pulmonary oedema is often seen in left-sided CHF but may also occur secondary to pulmonary hypertension. The oedema leads to an intrapulmonary short-circuit that induces hypoxaemia because the blood flowing through the pulmonary capillaries is poorly oxygenated due to impaired oxygen diffusion through the fluid-filled alveoli.

Patients with **pleural effusion** present with hypoventilation and hypoxaemia due to decreased lung volume and a tendency towards atelectasis.

Tachypnoea is a respiratory rate above 35–40 breaths per minute (bpm). Measurement of resting or sleeping respiratory rate is valuable for diagnosis of pulmonary oedema and for monitoring the response to treatment (in patients hospitalised for cardiogenic pulmonary oedema, this is the most sensitive and specific parameter for monitoring the evolution of the disease).

Respiratory rates above 35 bpm in patients with a prior diagnosis of left-sided heart disease suggest left-sided CHF. The owner should be instructed to monitor the respiratory rate at home and notify the veterinary surgeon as soon as possible of any increase to ensure prompt treatment. Dogs treated at home for CHF without pulmonary oedema have resting or sleeping respiratory rates below 30 bpm.

Dyspnoea is defined as breathing that is difficult or requires increased effort, and it is usually preceded and accompanied by tachypnoea. The patient appears short of breath and exerts significant effort to mobilise a larger volume of air, leading to anxiety and stress from feeling suffocated. Dyspnoea may appear with intense exercise (dyspnoea of exertion) or at rest with little physical activity. If it occurs at night while the patient is sleeping and awakens the patient, it is referred to as paroxysmal nocturnal dyspnoea. Orthopnoea is a respiratory sign in which the patient is reluctant to lie down and prefers to sit or stand; the patient assumes positions that aid in expanding the thorax and avoids any restriction of airflow into the lungs. These patients extend their necks, abduct their elbows, and dilate their nostrils in an effort to facilitate airflow into the airway. These signs generally indicate severe dyspnoea.

Cough is a common clinical sign in CHF patients. It may result from pulmonary oedema or compression of the trachea or left primary bronchus. This bronchial compression may result from a very dilated LA associated with tracheobronchomalacia. The cough may be a consequence of cardiac disease, but it can also result from tracheal collapse or chronic bronchitis.

Many patients with pulmonary oedema present only with increased vesicular sounds on auscultation, whereas crackles are more likely in patients with severe pulmonary oedema due to fluid in the airways. Breath sounds may be muffled in dogs with pleural effusion. Stridor, rhonchi, cough, and other pulmonary auscultation abnormalities may be related to an underlying respiratory disease.

Clinical signs of low cardiac output

The main causes of decreased cardiac output include bradyarrhythmias and tachyarrhythmias (supraventricular or ventricular tachycardia), severe pulmonary hypertension, cardiac tamponade, subaortic stenosis, or severe pulmonary stenosis with severe LV systolic dysfunction.

> Late-stage heart failure can decrease cardiac output, leading to weakness, lethargy, exercise intolerance, and syncope.

The physical examination reveals signs of low cardiac output: pale mucous membranes, prolonged capillary refill time, weak femoral pulse, hypotension, and tachycardia. The cardiovascular system's failure to maintain adequate tissue perfusion can induce cardiogenic shock, which includes other signs of hypoperfusion such as decreased urinary output and hyperlactataemia.

Weakness in CHF patients is connected to decreased blood flow to the muscle and hypoxaemia resulting from pulmonary oedema. Both factors decrease oxygen delivery and energy production in the muscle.

Exercise intolerance also results from insufficient oxygen supply to the tissues due to muscle hypoperfusion or low arterial blood oxygen content. These signs may be hidden in sedentary patients or those with unobservant owners, and they may go unnoticed until quite severe. The owner might also attribute these changes simply to ageing.

Syncope is a temporary loss of consciousness and posture due to a sudden decrease in cerebral blood flow. It often occurs with fainting, opisthotonus, front limb spasticity, and urination (due to sphincter relaxation); recovery is rapid. However, certain forms may be combined with seizures, so recovery may be slower. Episodes can occur during exertion or at rest, and they may be infrequent or occur several times per day.

General or systemic clinical signs

Dogs with chronic CHF tend to lose weight because of decreased body fat and muscle mass (cardiac cachexia). Muscle hypoperfusion, inflammatory phenomena, and oxidative stress are the main causes of weight loss. Right-sided CHF patients are more likely to suffer cachexia because ascites provides a feeling of fullness and delayed gastric emptying, which reduces appetite. In addition, systemic venous congestion can lead to pancreatic and intestinal oedema and lymphangectasia, which can result in malabsorption and protein-losing enteropathies. Usual CHF treatment (Chapter 4) can cause azotaemia, electrolyte disturbances like hyponatraemia and hypokalaemia, inappetence, and vomiting. Drugs such as digoxin (in toxicity cases) and amiodarone can also cause inappetence and vomiting. This process produces a negative energy balance and a deterioration of body condition that can be very severe.

LEFT-SIDED CHF

Diseases such as chronic mitral insufficiency, DCM, patent ductus arteriosus, VSD, and severe aortic regurgitation secondary to bacterial endocarditis are the most common causes of left-sided CHF in dogs. The main clinical signs include tachypnoea, dyspnoea, cough, fatigue, and exercise intolerance. Patients with severe pulmonary oedema show marked difficulty breathing and may cough and expel foam or pink fluid from the airways.

The most significant clinical sign of chronic mitral insufficiency is a systolic murmur, with a maximum intensity in the MV area. Systolic murmur can be detected from an early stage and generally intensifies as the disease progresses (intensity of the murmur reflects disease severity). The murmur is usually holosystolic and harsh, and it may be accompanied by a right apical murmur (tricuspid insufficiency or radiating mitral insufficiency murmur).

Dilated cardiomyopathy may involve a low-intensity systolic mitral insufficiency murmur or no murmur at all. Gallop rhythms and arrhythmias (generally atrial fibrillation and ventricular arrhythmias, potentially with pulsus alternans or pulse deficit) are also common auscultation findings in DCM. Dogs with patent ductus arteriosus have a continuous "machinery" murmur with maximum intensity in the left axillary region.

RIGHT-SIDED CHF

Pulmonary hypertension, heartworm, cardiac tamponade, tricuspid valve dysplasia, and cardiomyopathy are the most common causes of right-sided CHF in dogs. The most common clinical sign of right-sided CHF is abdominal distension due to ascites, but hepatomegaly, pleural effusion, and subcutaneous peripheral oedema (principally in hindlimbs) may also occur. Patients with atrial fibrillation and elevated heart rate often present with ascites. Dogs with pleural effusion and/or severe ascites may present with tachypnoea and dyspnoea.

The signs of systemic venous hypertension are jugular distension, jugular pulse, and positive hepatojugular reflux.

The most common cardiac auscultation findings in patients with pulmonary hypertensaion are a louder S2, a persistent split S2, and a holosystolic murmur of tricuspid regurgitation. Murmur intensity is variable and a murmur may go unnoticed in cases of pleural effusion.

Attenuated heart sounds and pulsus paradoxus are common findings in dogs with cardiac tamponade. Tricuspid valve dysplasia can cause a holosystolic murmur in the tricuspid auscultation area that can radiate to the left hemithorax. When the regurgitant orifice is very large, the flow is less turbulent, so the murmur is low-intensity (and sometimes even difficult to detect). Some patients with cardiomyopathy do not have murmurs.

FUNCTIONAL CLASSIFICATION

Functional classification systems categorise patients by severity of CHF and clinical signs. These systems are based on diagnostic tests and therapeutic protocols appropriate to each stage of the disease.

The three functional classification systems used in veterinary medicine are as follows:

- The modified New York Heart Association (NYHA) system.
- The International Small Animal Cardiac Health Council (ISACHC) system. In these two systems, the patient's functional class can change (to a less severe one) as the condition improves with treatment.
- The American College of Veterinary Internal Medicine (ACVIM) system, the newest one, is a veterinary adaptation of the American College of Cardiology/American Heart Association (ACC/AHA) classification system in the form of a consensus guide for diagnosis and treatment of canine chronic valvular disease. Patients remain in their initial functional class despite any improvement in clinical signs. In this system, a deterioration of condition changes the patient's functional class to one of greater severity. This system does not allow downgrading of functional class; it reflects the progression of cardiac disease and CHF, inspiring distinct recommendations for each stage of the disease.

Classification systems

Modified NYHA functional classification system

- Class 1: Patients with heart disease and no signs of CHF (even during exercise).
- Class 2: Patients with heart disease who show clinical signs (e.g. tachypnoea, dyspnoea, fatigue, weakness) only during exercise, not at rest.
- Class 3: Patients with heart disease who show clinical signs with ordinary physical activity.
- Class 4: patients with heart disease who show clinical signs even at rest.

ISACHC functional classification system

- Class 1: Patients with clinical evidence of cardiac disease but no CHF signs. Subclinical disease.
  - a: Patients without radiographic or echocardiographic evidence of remodelling (left cardiomegaly).
  - b: Patients with radiographic or echocardiographic evidence of remodelling.
- Class 2: Patients with cardiac disease who show mild or moderate signs of CHF (e.g. tachypnoea, dyspnoea, cough, exercise intolerance, fatigue, ascites, etc.).
- Class 3: Patients with advanced cardiac disease who show clinical signs of severe CHF (e.g. severe dyspnoea, marked exercise intolerance, signs of hypoperfusion, etc.). These can be divided into patients requiring hospitalisation and outpatients.

Table 1. Principal clinical signs of congestive heart failure.

Respiratory	Fluid retention	Low cardiac output	General or systemic
▸ Tachypnoea. ▸ Dyspnoea. ▸ Cough.	▸ Abdominal distension due to ascites. ▸ Oedema of the hindlimbs.	▸ Exercise intolerance: excessive fatigue while performing previously well-tolerated physical activities. ▸ Weakness. ▸ Fatigue. ▸ Syncope: fainting or transient loss of consciousness and posture.	▸ Weight loss. ▸ Decrease or loss of appetite: hyporexia or anorexia.

ACVIM functional classification for patients with chronic valvular disease

- Stage A: Patients with an increased risk of valvular disease who currently exhibit no structural or functional cardiac alterations (e.g. Cavalier King Charles Spaniel, Dachshund, Poodle, etc.).
- Stage B: Patients with subclinical disease. Dogs with evidence of valvular disease (e.g. patients with a murmur of mitral insufficiency) without signs of CHF.
  - B1: Patients without radiographic or echocardiographic evidence of remodelling (left cardiomegaly).
  - B2: Patients with radiographic or echocardiographic evidence of remodelling.
- Stage C: Patients who previously (prior to medical treatment) showed or currently show CHF signs related to structural heart disease. Those patients may be divided into:
  - Gravely ill patients who require intensive care in the hospital.
  - Patients with less severe signs who may be treated outpatient.
- Stage D: Patients with end-stage cardiac disease and clinical signs of CHF who have not responded adequately to standard treatment. Those patients require advanced or specialised treatment strategies to maintain a reasonable quality of life. They may be divided as follows:
  - Gravely ill patients who require intensive care in the hospital.
  - Patients with less severe signs who may receive outpatient care.

DIAGNOSIS

ECHOCARDIOGRAPHY

This chapter provides a guide to determine whether a patient's clinical signs (dyspnoea, ascites, etc.) are due to heart disease.

CHF may be diagnosed on an echocardiogram by the following steps:

- First, determine if echocardiographic signs compatible with pulmonary oedema, ascites, and/or pleural effusion are present.
- Next, look for significant cardiac remodelling from heart disease.
- Finally, demonstrate high ventricular end-diastolic pressures.

Each of these steps is important, as echocardiographic findings compatible with pulmonary oedema do not confirm that oedema is cardiogenic (e.g. heart disease may be mild and not account for the respiratory alteration). Signs of advanced heart disease associated with remodelling and high ventricular filling pressures are prerequisite findings for a CHF diagnosis.

Structural assessment of the left ventricle

Structural changes to the left ventricle (LV) representing adaptive responses to various pathologies can be classified as follows:

- Eccentric hypertrophy: ventricular dilation with a wall of normal thickness (pathologies inducing volume overload).
- Concentric hypertrophy: normal or decreased ventricular size with a thickened wall (pathologies inducing pressure overload).

Moderate to severe dilation is assessed in a long right parasternal view (covering the LV from the apex to the base) and short view (Table 1).

The ratio between LV wall thickness and diameter is as follows: normal LV diameter is 3 to 4 times the wall thickness. A larger diameter indicates dilation. A ratio of LV diastolic diameter to aortic root diameter that is greater than 3 indicates a high risk of CHF in patients with mitral insufficiency. Reference tables of linear LV dimensions (M-mode), both for specific breeds and by weight independent of breed, are available (Fig. 1). Use breed-specific values when available and values by weight otherwise. Reference values may be linear or allometric, but the allometric scale is most sensitive for identifying mild to moderate LV dilation.

Table 1. Characteristics of a normal and dilated left ventricle (LV) in long and short ultrasound views.

	Normal LV	Dilated LV
Long view	Conical shape, with straight interventricular septum (IVS) at end-diastole.	Spherical shape, with IVS curved towards right ventricle and rounded apex (Fig. 2).
Short view	Rounded; endocardial surface is smooth and regular, interrupted only by papillary muscles. Echo-free ventricle, except for the mitral valve. Mushroom-shaped internal cavity (papillary muscles).	Mushroom shape is not discernible (Fig. 3).

Assessing left ventricle systolic function

Assessment of systolic function is critical, since LV global systolic dysfunction is a prerequisite to diagnose cardiomyopathy as well as an indicator of progression and severity of cardiac diseases.

> Keep in mind that patients with relatively normal systolic function may have CHF, and patients with mild to moderate global systolic dysfunction may lack clinical signs of congestion.

In cases of myocardial insufficiency, the ventricle may be dilated, with marked global hypocontractility (decreased systolic excursion from the septum and free wall) of varying degrees.

The LV end-systolic linear dimension in M-mode should be compared to the reference values for the patient's weight. A value higher than the maximum for the patient's weight suggests global systolic dysfunction.

Fractional shortening and ejection fraction are two of the most useful and most commonly employed parameters to assess LV systolic function.

Fractional shortening

Fractional shortening is a percentage that expresses the change or decrease between LV end-diastolic and end-systolic dimensions. Measurements of the LV are obtained in M-mode for this calculation (Figs. 4 and 5), using a short right parasternal view at the level of the papillary muscles or chordae tendinae, placing the cursor perpendicular to the LV between the papillary muscles. Values above 30 % are considered normal. Fractional shortening is calculated with the following formula:

$$\text{Fractional shortening} = \frac{EDD - ESD}{EDD}$$

EDD = end-diastolic dimension ESD = end-systolic dimension.

In diseases with LV dilation, such as mitral insufficiency, the fractional shortening may fall within the reference range despite the presence of heart failure.

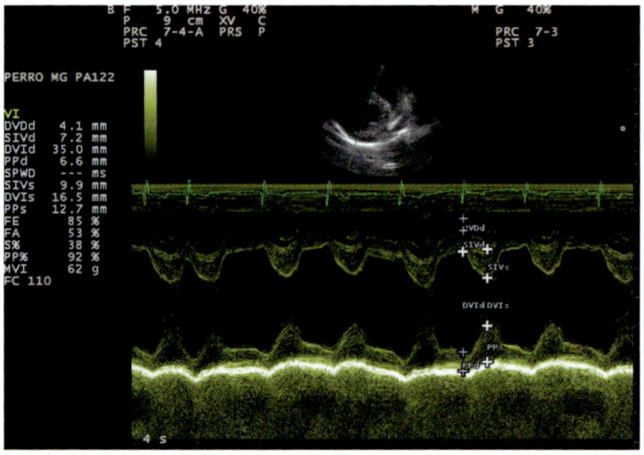

Figure 1. Left ventricular M-mode echocardiogram in a dog with severe left ventricular eccentric hypertrophy secondary to mitral insufficiency.

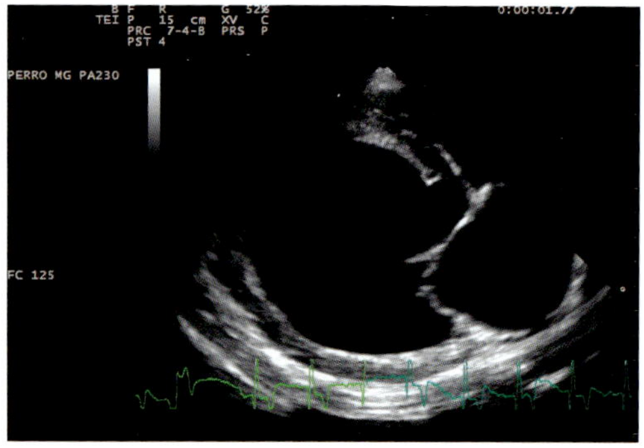

Figure 2. Severe eccentric hypertrophy in a patient with patent ductus arteriosus. Long right parasternal view.

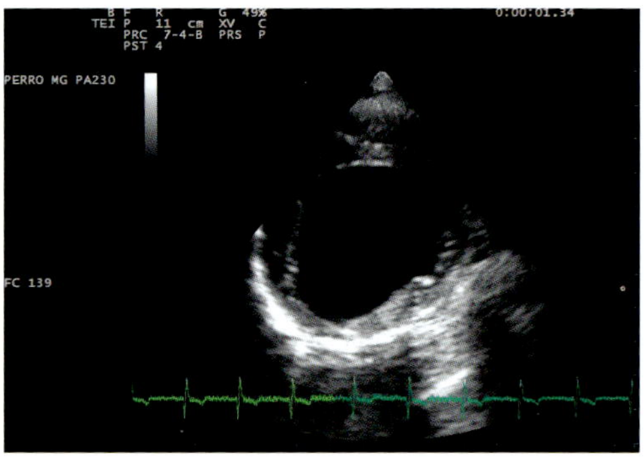

Figure 3. Left ventricular dilation in a patient with dilated cardiomyopathy. Short right parasternal view.

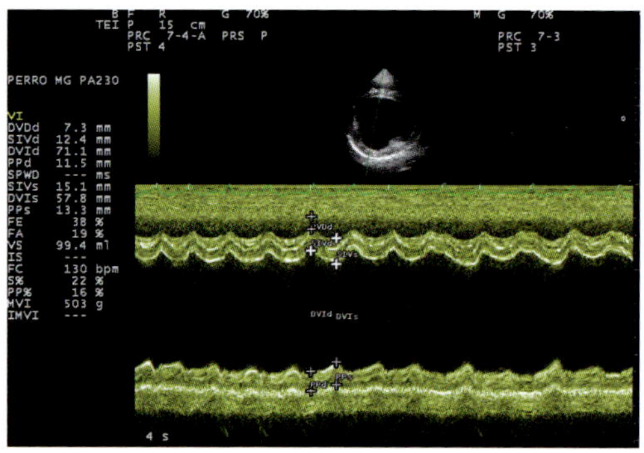

Figure 4. Left ventricular M-mode echocardiogram. Patient with dilated cardiomyopathy and moderate to severe left ventricular global systolic dysfunction (fractional shortening of 19 %).

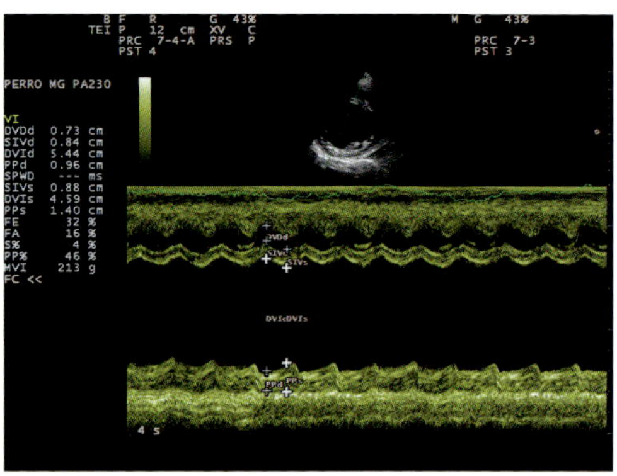

Figure 5. Left ventricular M-mode echocardiogram. Patient with severe left ventricular global systolic dysfunction secondary to severe mitral insufficiency (fractional shortening of 16 %).

Ejection fraction

The ejection fraction is a percentage that expresses the change between LV end-diastolic and end-systolic volumes. The images needed to calculate the LV volumes may be obtained in M-mode (Teicholz method) or B-mode (modified Simpson's rule or area-length method). The ejection fraction in B-mode can be obtained using a right parasternal long-axis four-chamber view (Fig. 6) or an apical four-chamber view. Delineate the endocardial border and the ventricular length (from the plane of the mitral annulus to the apex) at end-diastole and end-systole. Values above 50 % are considered normal.

Structural assessment of the left atrium

Left atrial (LA) dilation is the classic remodelling that the heart undergoes as a result of the various pathologies that induce LA volume or pressure overload. Identifying it is critical to CHF diagnosis, given that an animal with LA dilation carries a high risk of developing CHF.

> The vast majority of patients with left-sided CHF have moderate to severe LA dilation.

Although rare, pulmonary oedema may arise without LA dilation when an acute rupture of chordae tendinae occurs; this leads to severe mitral regurgitation in a patient lacking atrial dilation.

Atrial measurement in M-mode is not recommended in dogs because the placement of the M-mode cursor across the atrial appendage or at the junction between the appendage and the body of the atrium underestimates atrial size. Atrial diameter is usually measured in B-mode in a short right parasternal view at the level of the heart base, showing the sinus of Valsalva and the atrial appendage. It should be measured at the end of systole (point of maximum atrial distension), seen in the first cine-loop frame right when the aortic valve closes. The ratio between the left atrial diameter and the aortic diameter (LA:aorta ratio) should always be calculated (Fig. 7).

- The aortic diameter is usually measured by tracing a line from the inner edge of the commissure between the left coronary sinus and the non-coronary sinus to the inner edge of the middle of the right coronary sinus.
- The LA is measured by tracing a line parallel to the aorta and placing the ends of the line on the inner edges of the atrial walls.

An LA:aorta ratio up to 1.5 is considered normal; values up to 1.9 represent mild dilation; up to 2.2 is considered moderate, and higher values are severe.

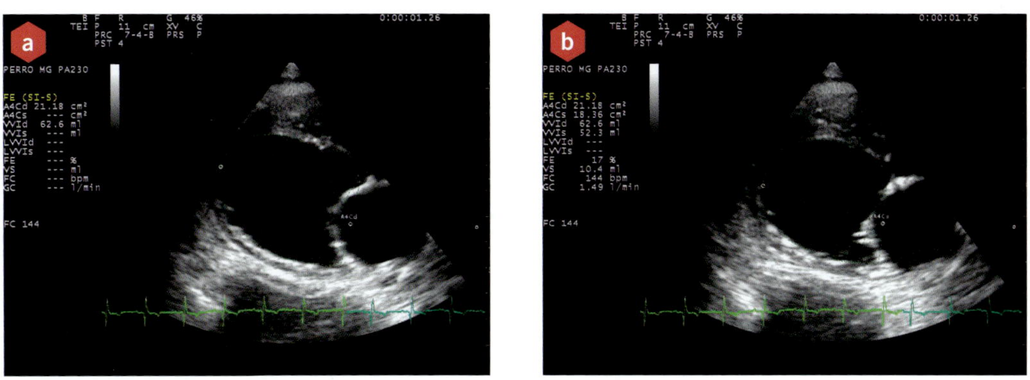

Figure 6. Ejection fraction computed by modified Simpson method on a long right parasternal view. Patient with dilated cardiomyopathy and severe left ventricular global systolic dysfunction (ejection fraction of 17 %).
(a) Left ventricle at end-diastole, and (b) at end-systole.

Estimation of left ventricular diastolic filling pressure

Doppler echocardiographic indices are used to estimate volume status and LV end-diastolic pressures, allowing early recognition of CHF and objective monitoring of the treatment response.

Adequate diastolic function involves good ventricular filling with normal LA, venous, and pulmonary capillary pressures. The integrity of this function depends on several factors: ventricular distensibility, active myocardial relaxation, atrial contraction, and mean LA pressure. Left ventricular filling is assessed in terms of transmitral diastolic flow and involves measuring E and A wave velocities, the E:A ratio, the isovolumetric relaxation time (IVRT), and the E wave deceleration time (DT).

Transmitral flow comprises two phases: the rapid or early LV filling phase (result of active myocardial relaxation, represented by the E wave) and the late filling phase (result of atrial contraction, represented by the A wave). Under normal conditions, the first phase constitutes 80 % of ventricular filling.

The images used to evaluate diastolic function are obtained in the apical four-chamber view, with the 4 mm pulsed Doppler sample placed between the tips of the MV leaflets during maximal opening. The E and A waves are seen above the baseline. Deceleration time is the time from the peak E wave velocity to baseline, and it reflects the speed at which pressures equilibrate between the ventricle and atrium. Under normal flow, E wave velocity is greater than A wave velocity, the E:A ratio is between one and two, and the maximum E velocity is 0.6 to 1.1 m/s (Fig. 8).

Isovolumetric relaxation time begins with the closure of the AV and ends with the opening of the MV. During this period, the LV volume does not change. Active myocardial relaxation initiates isovolumetric relaxation, the interval in which the LV pressure falls below the LA pressure, inducing the MV to open (Fig. 9).

The spectral tissue Doppler tracing of the mitral annulus comprises an Sa wave that represents myocardial systolic velocity, an Ea wave that represents myocardial diastolic velocity, and an Aa wave that represents atrial contraction. These images are obtained in the apical four-chamber view, with the sample volume (4–6 mm) placed at the lateral mitral annulus. Normally, the Ea wave is larger than the Aa wave (Fig. 10).

Various factors affect the transmitral flow pattern: heart rate and rhythm, active myocardial relaxation, atrial contraction, and mean LA pressure.

When the heart rate is high, both filling phases may be superimposed and fuse into one wave. The lack of a second diastolic phase means the A wave is absent, as is seen during atrial fibrillation or atrial standstill. During atrial fibrillation, the irregular rhythm alters the diastolic time and E wave velocity (Fig. 11). Left atrial pressure or volume overload increases E wave velocity and causes earlier MV opening with shortened IVRT.

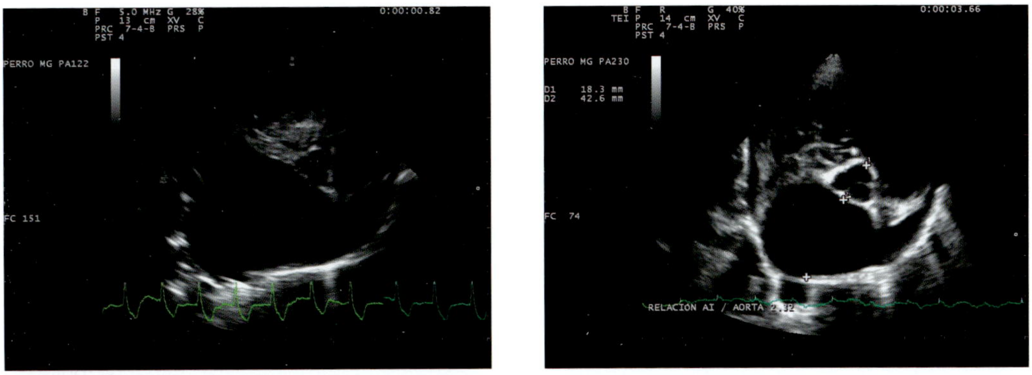

Figure 7. Severe left atrial dilation in two mitral insufficiency patients.

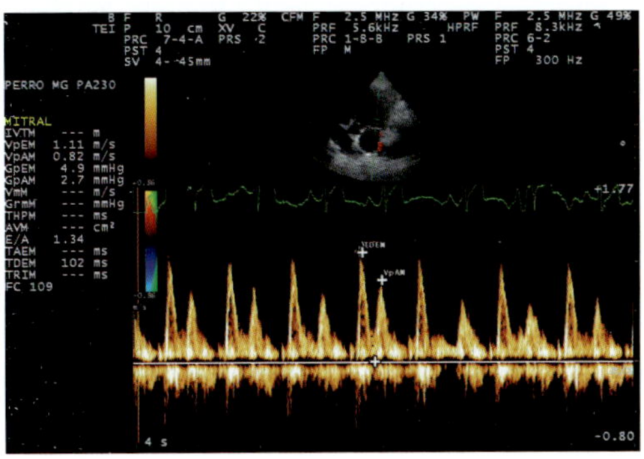

Figure 8. Normal transmitral flow tracing.

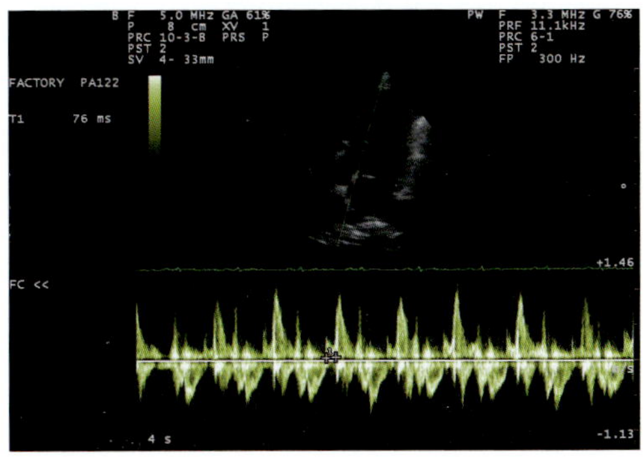

Figure 9. Isovolumetric relaxation time (IVRT) measurement. IVRT measurement is based on an apical five-chamber view, with the sample volume placed between the left ventricular outflow tract and the mitral valve to capture left ventricular systolic flow and transmitral diastolic flow; this marks the end of systolic flow and the start of diastolic flow.

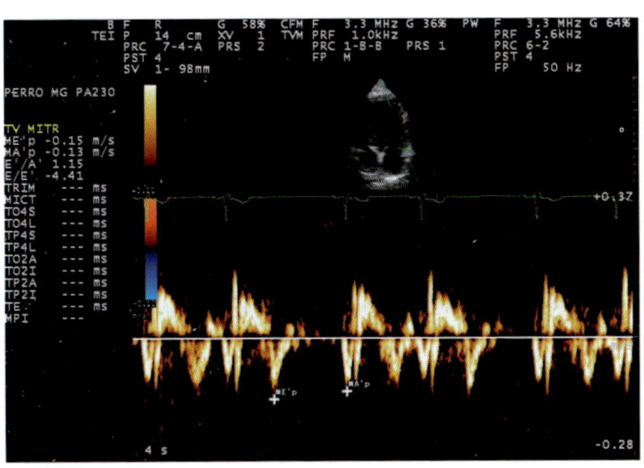

Figure 10. Normal spectral tissue Doppler tracing of lateral mitral annulus. Systolic motion is above baseline, while diastolic waves are under baseline.

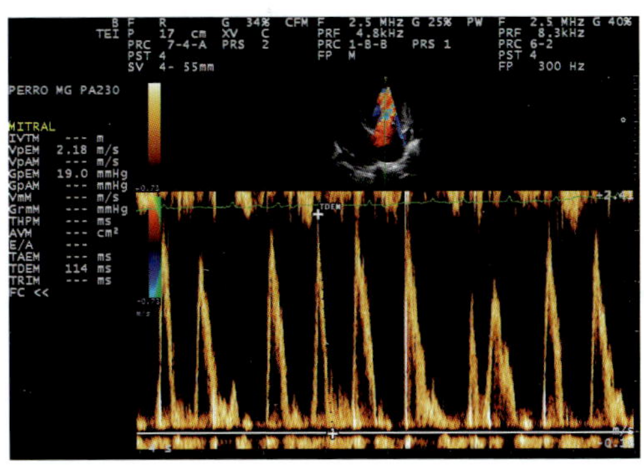

Figure 11. Transmitral flow in a patient with atrial fibrillation. E waves are rapid and inconsistent; A waves are absent.

Three grades of diastolic dysfunction exist: impaired myocardial relaxation, pseudonormalisation, and restrictive filling.

- Diastolic dysfunction due to **impaired myocardial relaxation** is the lowest grade of dysfunction (grade 1); it is a normal physiological variant in dogs older than 10 years and in asymptomatic dogs with mild cardiac disease (Fig. 12). It is characterised by a decrease in E wave velocity, an increase in the A wave, an E:A ratio less than one, and an increase in IVRT and in DT of the E wave (Fig. 13a). In tissue Doppler of the lateral mitral annulus, Ea velocity is lower than the Aa velocity (Fig. 13b). Alteration of myocardial relaxation decreases transvalvular flow and E wave velocity, and atrial contraction compensates for the filling deficit during the first phase by increasing the flow and A wave velocity. A decrease in E velocity with an increase in the A wave may be observed in patients with decreased preload and in patients with severe pulmonary hypertension. This degree of diastolic dysfunction rules out elevated ventricular filling pressures or CHF.
- **Pseudonormalisation** is a more severe grade of dysfunction (grade 2) that results from fundamentally impaired relaxation, but LA volume or pressure overload alters the transmitral flow such that it appears normal. The LA pressure rise results in an increased E wave velocity, which had previously decreased due to impaired relaxation, and the MV opens more quickly, decreasing the IVRT. This combination of factors pseudonormalises the transmitral flow and produces an E wave of normal or increased velocity, an E:A ratio between one and two, and normal DT and IVRT. However, tissue Doppler of the mitral annulus shows an underlying relaxation impairment, with an Ea wave velocity below that of the Aa wave and an Ea:Aa ratio less than one (Fig. 14). Patients with grade 2 dysfunction are at greater risk of pulmonary oedema, so in these cases it is important to check if the LV end-diastolic pressure is increased. Elevated E:Ea and E:IVRT ratios indicate high ventricular filling pressures.

In summary, a high E wave velocity (>1.3 m/s), associated with a low Ea wave velocity or a shortened IVRT, is compatible with left-sided CHF (Fig. 15).

- **Restricted ventricular filling, referred to as a restrictive pattern,** is the most advanced stage of diastolic dysfunction (grade 3) and is seen in severe disease as a decrease in myocardial distensibility and LA volume or pressure overload. In this stage, ventricular filling occurs with high pressures and atrial emptying is incomplete. This pattern is characterised by an elevated E velocity, a decreased A velocity, E:A ratio >2 (Fig. 16a), and decreased DT and IVRT. Increased LA pressures raise E wave velocities and decrease IVRT. The decreased distensibility means pressures equalise more quickly between the left chambers, decreasing the DT (<80 m/s). The high early ventricular diastolic pressures restrict late filling, decreasing the A wave velocity. The spectral tissue Doppler of the mitral annulus may be attenuated, which is why the E:Ea (Fig. 16b) and E:IVRT ratios are relevant to estimating ventricular filling pressures. An E:Ea ratio below 11.5 in dogs with mitral insufficiency or below 9 in dogs with cardiomyopathy are highly suggestive of left-sided CHF. Patients with this degree of diastolic dysfunction often present with pulmonary oedema or are at high risk of developing it.

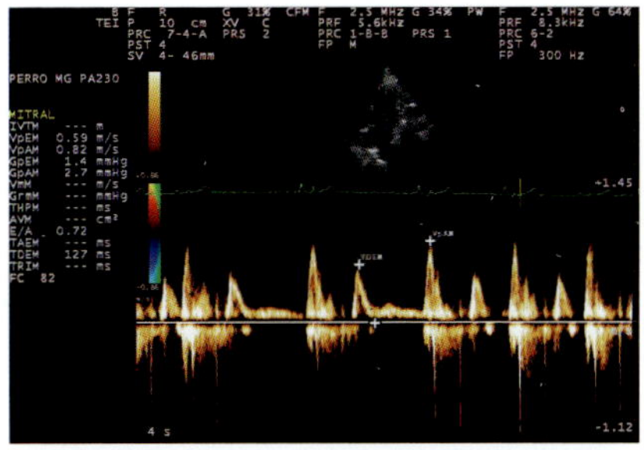

Figure 12. Diastolic dysfunction due to impaired myocardial relaxation. Normal physiological variant in a dog over 10 years old without cardiomyopathy.

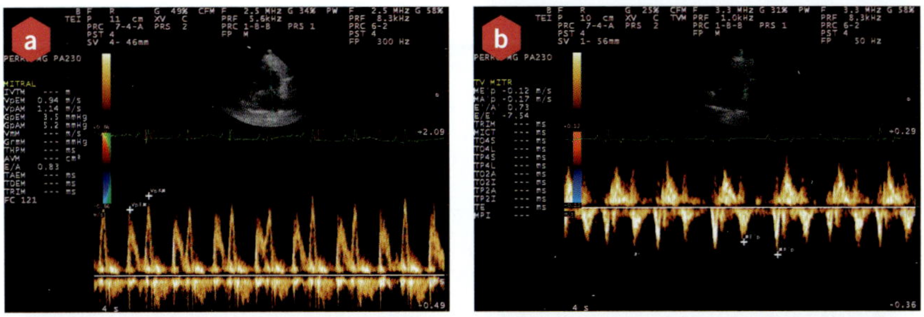

Figure 13. Diastolic dysfunction due to impaired myocardial relaxation. Transmitral flow (a) and tissue Doppler (b) of lateral mitral annulus.

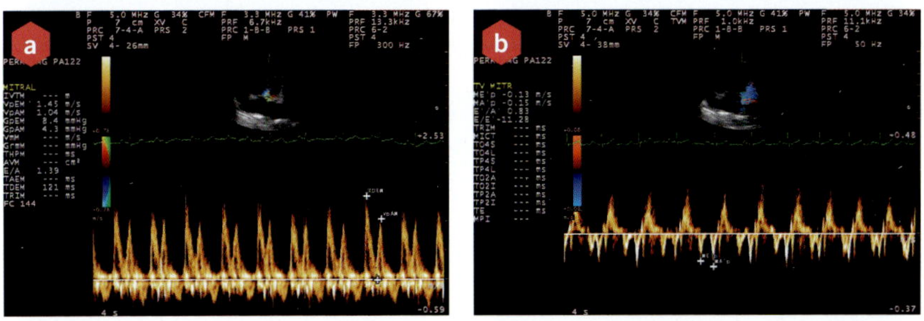

Figure 14. Grade 2 diastolic dysfunction. Transmitral flow is pseudonormalised (a) and tissue Doppler demonstrates impaired relaxation (b).

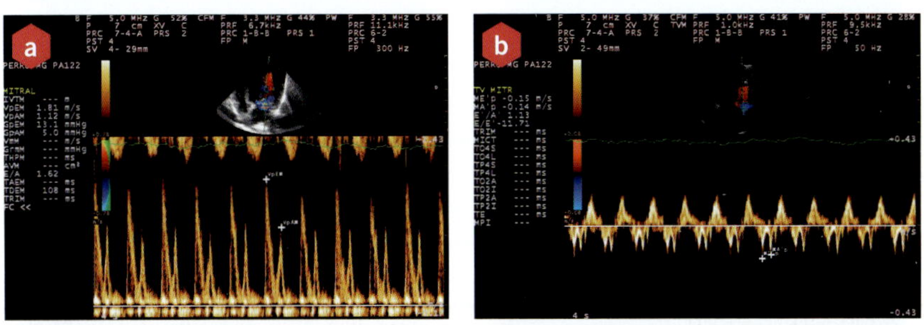

Figure 15. Pseudonormalisation. (a) E waves are rapid, and (b) the E:Ea ratio is increased (11,71). Findings suggestive of left-sided congestive heart failure.

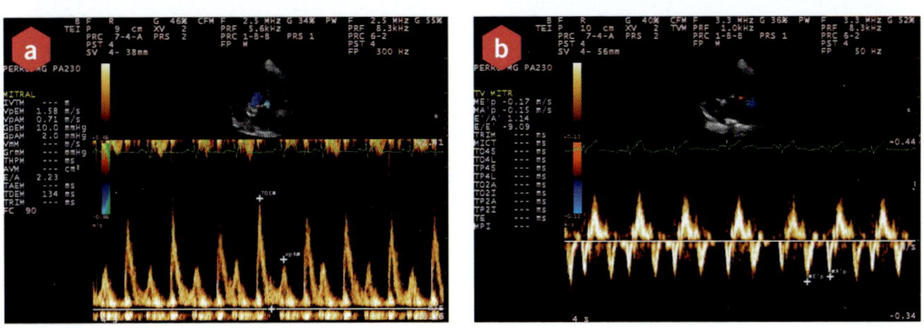

Figure 16. Diastolic dysfunction due to restrictive ventricular filling. Transmitral flow (a) and tissue Doppler (b).

Ultrasound findings in left-sided CHF

Lung ultrasound is rapidly becoming a test of choice for assessing critically dyspnoeic patients. Microconvex, sector (phased array), or linear transducers may be used. The transducer should be placed with the ultrasound beam oriented horizontally (although it can also be oriented vertically) with a sector depth of 4–6 cm. A lung ultrasound protocol by G. Lisciandro called Vet Blue (an acronym of Bedside Lung Ultrasound in Emergency/Exam) is available for patients with dyspnoea. In this protocol, the transducer is placed on four regions of the thoracic wall:

- Caudodorsal lung lobe region, in the upper third of the thorax between the eighth and ninth intercostal space (approximately dorsal to the xiphoid).
- Perihilar lung lobe region, in the middle third of the thorax between the sixth and seventh intercostal space.
- Middle lung lobe region, in the lower third of the thorax between the fourth and fifth intercostal space (around the heart). Cranial lung lobe region, in the lower third of the thorax between the second and third intercostal space (cranial to the heart).

Healthy lung

Aiming the beam horizontally in the near field provides a transverse section of the ribs, which appear rounded and hyperechoic and cast an acoustic shadow (although sector [phased array] transducers do not always permit identification of the ribs). The near field shows hypoechoic soft tissue between the ribs, corresponding to subcutaneous tissue and intercostal muscles, and, underneath, a hyperechoic, horizontal pulmonary–pleural line. Normal lungs show a glide sign, the result of movement between the parietal and visceral pleura that coincides with the motion of breathing and rules out a pleural space-occupying lesion. A-lines, which are air reverberation artefacts from contact between soft tissue and healthy lung, are also observed. These are hyperechoic, horizontal lines parallel to the pulmonary–pleural line that start below it and repeat to the deepest parts of the sector (Fig. 17).

Pulmonary oedema/interstitial syndrome

Patients with pulmonary oedema show an ultrasound pattern compatible with interstitial syndrome: a glide sign and a comet tail, or B-line, artefact. These are hyperechoic bands or lines that extend vertically from the pulmonary-pleural line across the sector (to the far field) and move along with the lung glide (Fig. 18). This pattern appears when the periphery of the lung lobes is affected. Differential diagnoses for interstitial syndrome include pulmonary oedema (cardiogenic or noncardiogenic), pulmonary contusion, fibrosis and pneumonia.

The more B-lines appear, the more severe the oedema:

- One, two, or three B-lines: small amount (Fig. 19).
- >3 B-lines: when more than three lines appear but they are individually identifiable (Fig. 20).
- A full white screen (hyperechoic) without identifiable A- or B-lines is considered as corresponding to 10 B-lines and indicates very severe oedema (Fig. 21).

Others

Pleural effusion is observed as an anechoic space that separates the lung lobes from the chest wall and diaphragm; lung tissue appears to flap in the effusion (Fig. 22).

Lung lobe consolidation is characterised by hypoechoic areas (tissue sign) crossed by hyperechoic lines representing air-filled airways.

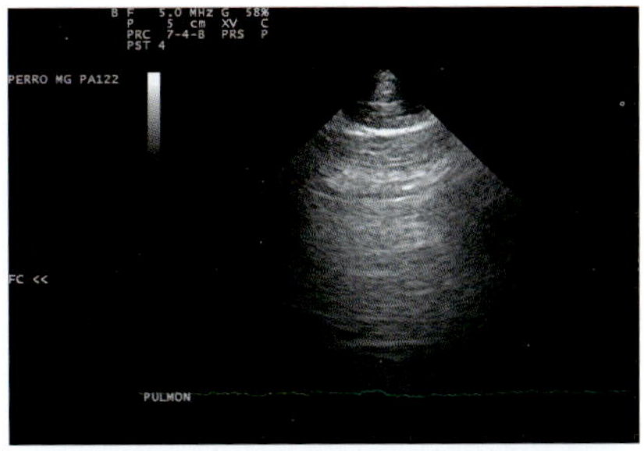

Figure 17. Normal lung. The pleuropulmonary line (glide sign) and A-lines are visible.

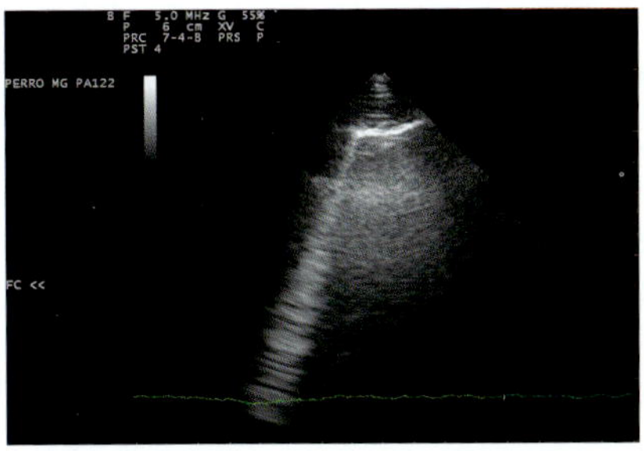

Figure 18. Interstitial syndrome. A B-line, or comet tail, artefact is seen.

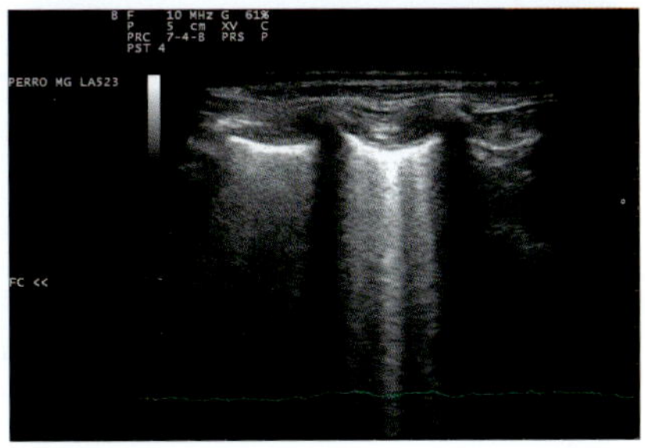

Figure 19. Two B-lines are visible in an intercostal space. Patients with cardiogenic pulmonary oedema.

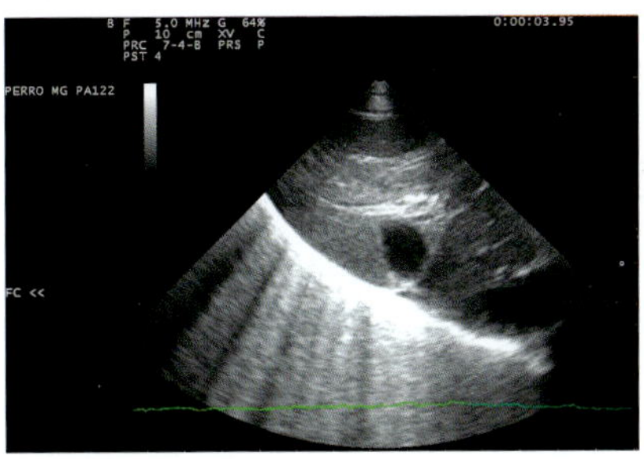

Figure 20. Subcostal view. The near field shows the liver and a hyperechoic line between the diaphragm and lung, the point of origin of many B-lines in a patient with severe pulmonary oedema secondary to dilated cardiomyopathy.

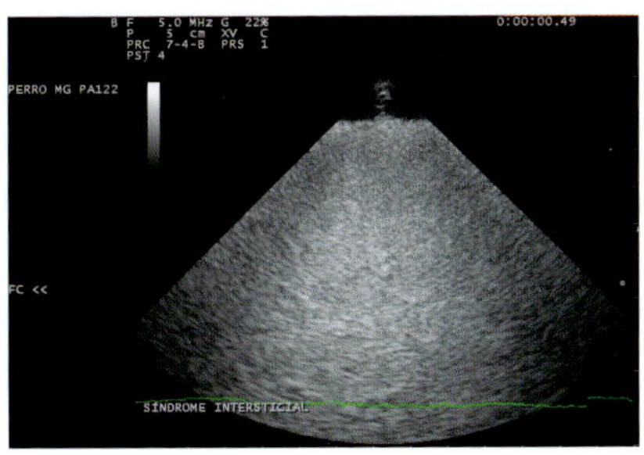

Figure 21. The entire field is hyperechoic, without identifiable A waves. Findings compatible with severe pulmonary oedema.

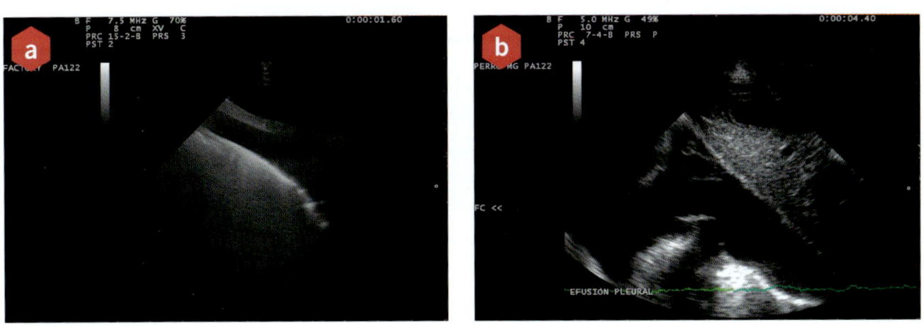

Figure 22. Pleural effusion from an intercostal (a) and subcostal (b) view.

Structural assessment of the right ventricle and atrium

The right ventricular free wall (RVFW) and the triangular ventricle are visible in the upper part of the image on a long right parasternal view. The RVFW:LVFW ratio should be between 0.33 and 0.5. Diseases with higher systolic wall stress due to increased intraventricular pressure, such as pulmonary hypertension or stenosis, tend to have a higher ratio.

The normal ratio between RV and LV diastolic diameters is less than 0.5. Right ventricular dilation causes an increase in this ratio; between 0.5 and 1 is considered mild to moderate, and above 1 is considered severe.

Pulmonary stenosis gives rise to RV concentric hypertrophy in which wall thickness increases without chamber dilation. In these cases, the interventricular septum (IVS) may hypertrophy similarly to the RVFW. Right ventricular dilation is characteristic of disorders of volume overload such as tricuspid dysplasia or RV arrhythmogenic cardiomyopathy. Patients with pulmonary hypertension may also have ventricular dilation, but it is associated with greater RVFW thickening (Fig. 23).

In cases of RV volume or pressure overload, the IVS may be displaced towards the LV, as a result of the higher RV end-diastolic pressure (exceeding that of the LV). This haemodynamic alteration produces a septal flattening sign (Fig. 24), which appears in the short view at the level of the papillary muscles or chordae

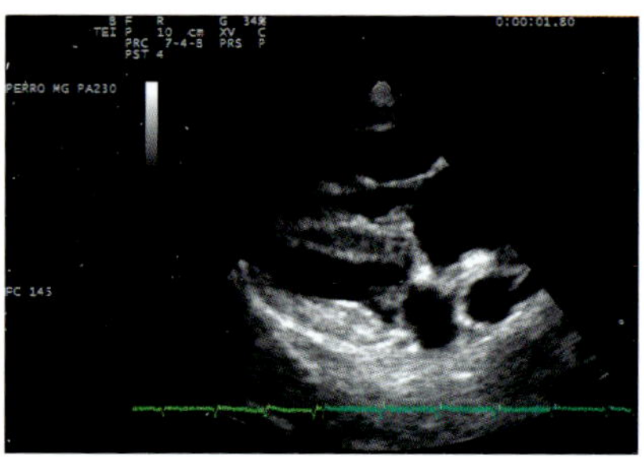

Figure 23. Severe right ventricular eccentric hypertrophy in a dog with pulmonary hypertension. Long right parasternal view.

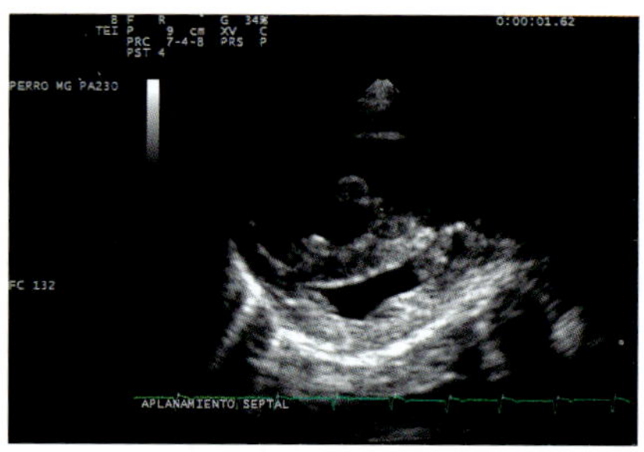

Figure 24. Severe right ventricular eccentric hypertrophy with septal flattening in a patient with pulmonary hypertension. Short right parasternal view.

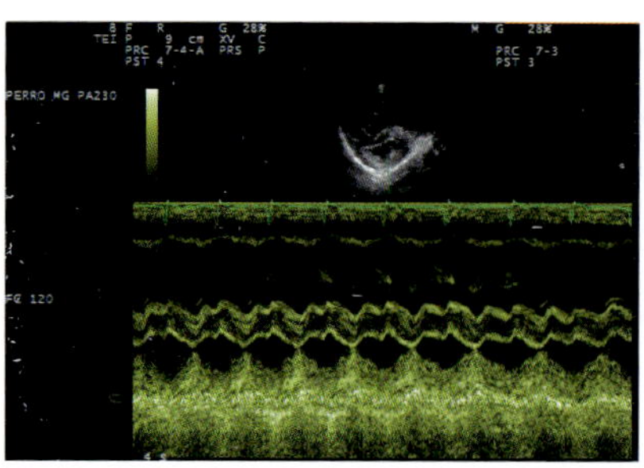

Figure 25. Paradoxical motion of the interventricular septum.

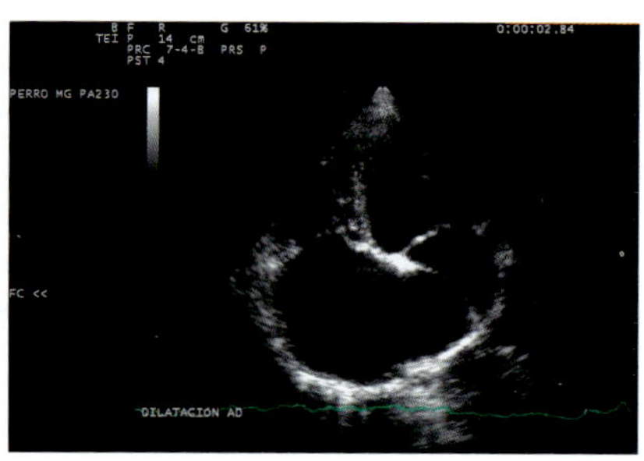

Figure 26. Significant right atrial dilation. Apical four-chamber view.

tendinae. This abnormal IVS motion seen in M-mode is referred to as paradoxical motion of the IVS (Fig. 25).

Right atrial (RA) size may be assessed in a right long parasternal four-chamber view or an apical four-chamber view. The atrial sizes can be subjectively compared. The LA is usually slightly larger than or the same size as the RA. When dilated, the RA is larger than the LA, and the interatrial septum can be seen curving towards the left side (Fig. 26).

Ultrasound findings in right-sided CHF

Dogs with right-sided CHF may present with ascites and/or pleural effusion. In patients with abdominal distension, the first step is an ultrasound to confirm the presence of free abdominal fluid. The fluid accumulating in the abdomen in CHF is typically an anechoic transudate without suspended echogenicities.

The animal should be placed in right lateral recumbency for the echocardiogram; moreover, this position is more comfortable than dorsal recumbency for a patient with ascites.

With severe ascites, the fluid is easy to identify. When the abdominal distension is not severe, the transducer may be placed at specific spots to optimise fluid detection: the subcostal view (placing the transducer just caudal to the xiphoid) reveals anechoic areas between the diaphragm and the liver, between the liver lobes (Fig. 27), between the liver and the stomach, and around the gallbladder. In the caudal abdomen, a dependent area can be assessed at the level of the urinary bladder apex. Anechoic areas may appear in the left lateral abdomen between the spleen and the abdominal wall, or the spleen and the left kidney, and in the right lateral abdomen between the cranial pole of the right kidney and the liver.

Evaluate patients with ascites for signs of congestion. Systemic venous hypertension implicates a congestive cause of ascites, including right-sided CHF or Budd–Chiari syndrome (resulting from a partial or complete obstruction of venous return between the hepatic veins and RA). Thrombosis of the caudal vena cava (CaVC), a tumour in the cavity of the RA or lumen of the CaVC, or any tumour that compromises the CaVC can give rise to this syndrome. Although examination of the jugular vein

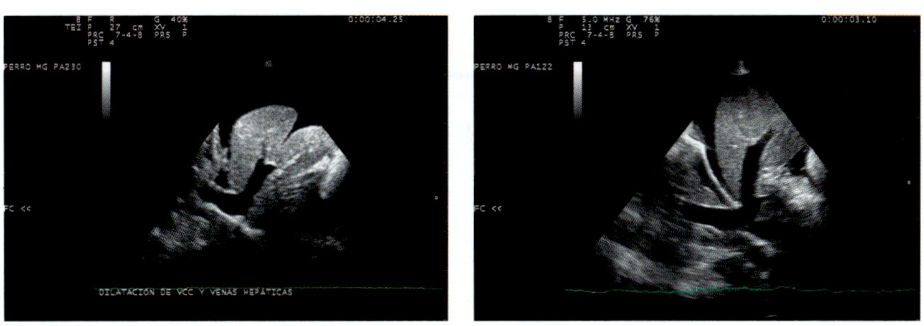

Figure 27. Subcostal views of peritoneal effusion between the liver lobes and between the liver and diaphragm. Dilation of the hepatic veins and caudal vena cava are also visible.

and identification of a jugular pulse or distension has been the noninvasive method of choice to estimate systemic venous pressure, ultrasound examination of the hepatic veins and CaVC is now a very sensitive noninvasive method.

Hepatic veins

The hepatic veins (HVs) are anechoic tubular structures that run from the peripheral hepatic parenchyma to the hilar region (near the diaphragm) and can be seen entering the CaVC. Their diameter increases as they approach the CaVC and decreases towards the periphery. Their walls are hypoechoic to the portal vein walls. The best views are right dorsal subcostal and intercostal. Systemic venous hypertension leads to HV distension (Fig. 28). If distension is severe, the increase in diameter is apparent and easily recognised; portal vein diameters should be used for reference, as they are similar to those of HVs. In case of HV dilation, their diameters greatly exceed the portal vein diameter.

Caudal vena cava

Caudal vena cava (CaVC) diameter varies cyclically with respiration. It decreases with inspiration, when the intrathoracic pressure falls, systemic venous return increases and the CaVC empties more fully. During expiration, CaVC diameter increases as systemic venous return decreases.

To estimate central venous pressure (CVP), assess the portion of the CaVC closest to the diaphragm on a long subcostal view (Figs. 29 and 30) in M-mode, placing the cursor perpendicular to the part of the CaVC with the most variable diameter. This mode measures the expiratory and inspiratory diameters, so the percentage of inspiratory collapse can be determined:

- 100 % inspiratory collapse: corresponds to a non-dilated CaVC, compatible with a CVP of 0 to 5 mmHg.
- Between 50 and 100 %: CVP is estimated to be between 6 and 10 mmHg.
- Below 50 %: CVP is likely between 11 and 15 mmHg (Fig. 31).
- Absence of collapse (0 %): corresponds to a dilated CaVC and indicates a CVP above 15 mmHg, associated with dilated HVs and ascites. Generally speaking, ascites associated with a dilated CaVC (with absent or minimal inspiratory collapse) and dilated HVs indicates systemic venous hypertension and a congestive cause of ascites.

> The HVs and CaVC may be distended in situations such as fluid overload (due to excess intravenous fluids), sedation with drugs such as alpha-2 agonists, and positive pressure ventilation.

Pericardial effusion and cardiac tamponade

Pericardial effusion appears as an anechoic area around the heart between the epicardium and parietal pericardium (pericardial sac). The contour of the pericardial sac is smooth and rounded around the heart (Fig. 32). If a pleural effusion is also present, the pericardial sac thickness can be assessed using the contrast that the effusion provides on either side of the sac.

The pericardial sac is most strongly adhered to the epicardium at the heart base, so effusions are not always seen around the atria. If the effusion is extensive, the atria can be seen floating in the fluid, along with a swinging motion of the heart. For small-volume effusions, a small anechoic area is detected behind the LVFW or around the apex. A decrease in

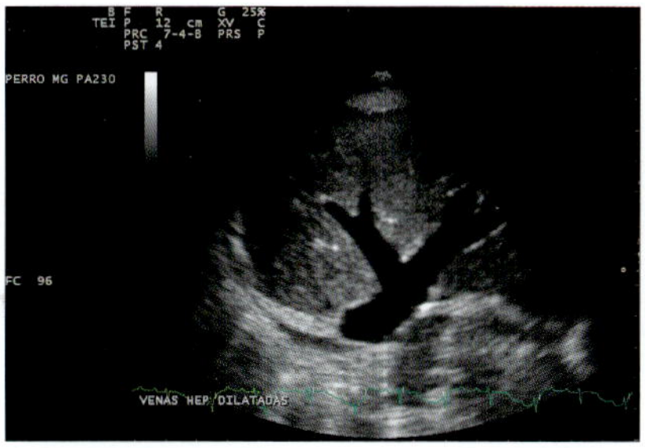

Figure 28. Dilation of the hepatic veins. Short view.

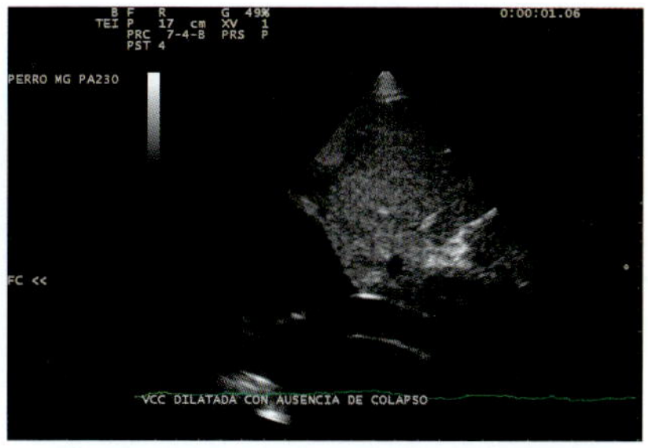

Figure 29. Dilation of the caudal vena cava without inspiratory collapse. Patient with pleural effusion.

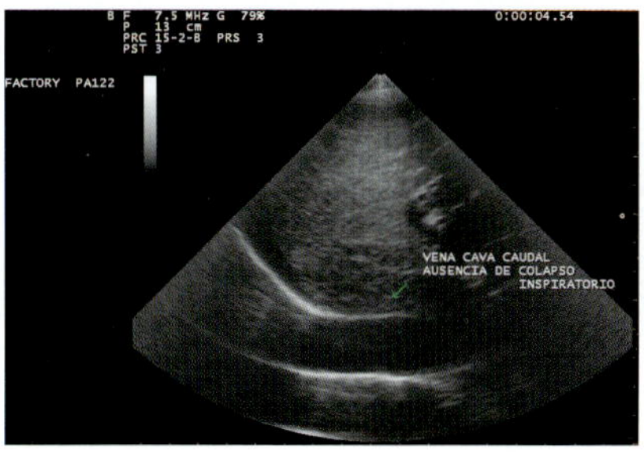

Figure 30. Dilation of the caudal vena cava without inspiratory collapse. Patient with pleural effusion.

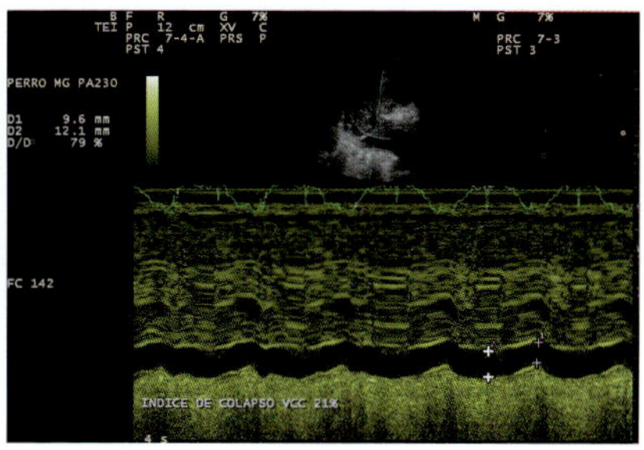

Figure 31. M-mode ultrasound of the caudal vena cava for calculating the caval index. Patient with a caval index of 21 %, compatible with a central venous pressure of 11–15 mmHg.

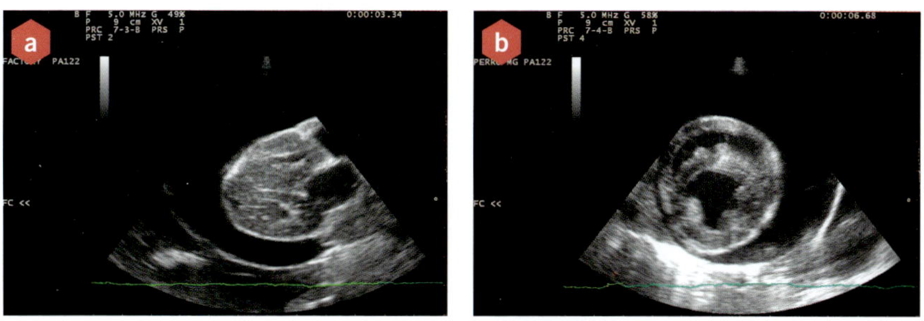

Figure 32. Extensive pericardial effusion. Long (a) and short (b) right parasternal views.

ventricular diameter and pseudohypertrophy may be subjectively noted.

Right atrial collapse is a sensitive and specific sign of cardiac tamponade (Fig. 33). Right ventricular collapse may also be observed.

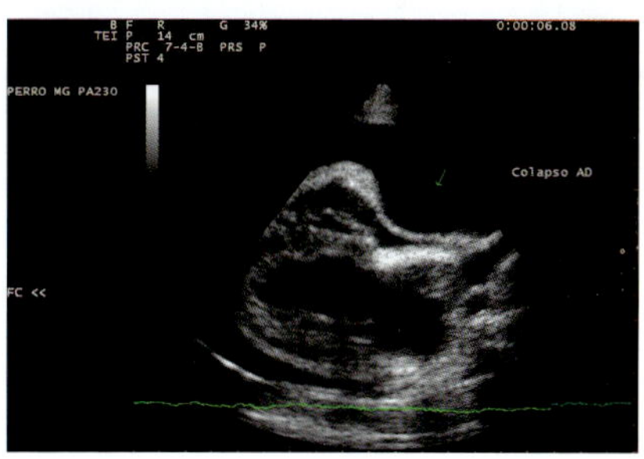

Figure 33. Right atrial collapse in a dog with cardiac tamponade.

BIOMARKERS

A biomarker is a substance released by a particular tissue that can be identified and measured in plasma. In veterinary cardiology, the most useful biomarkers are B-type natriuretic peptide (BNP) and cardiac troponin I (cTnI). Cardiac troponin I is useful for detecting myocardial lesions (ischaemia, necrosis, or inflammation) and establishing the risk of mortality. Values above 0.025 ng/ml correlate with a higher mortality in dogs with mitral insufficiency. B-type natriuretic peptide is released as a result of increased ventricular and atrial wall stress. It is useful for determining the origin of respiratory signs (tachypnoea, dyspnoea, and cough) and establishing the prognosis. It helps to differentiate whether respiratory signs are due to CHF or to primary respiratory disease. It may be most useful in emergency situations, when no X-ray or ultrasound equipment is available, when the results of those tests are inconclusive, or when the patient is not able to tolerate those tests. Patients with pulmonary hypertension secondary to respiratory disease may have elevated BNP, which complicates interpretation of the results. Values above 1400 pmol/l indicate a higher likelihood of CHF, and it is unlikely with values below 900 pmol/l. Values above 1500 pmol/l indicate a higher risk of mortality from cardiac causes.

RADIOGRAPHY

Thoracic radiographs are useful for detecting cardiomegaly, but they are imprecise, particularly in mild to moderate cases. Various factors including thoracic conformation, age, phase of respiration, cardiac cycle, and pericardial fat, can alter the cardiac silhouette. This variability is one reason why radiographs are imprecise for detecting generalised cardiomegaly and dilation of a particular chamber. Echocardiography is a much more precise test for chamber dilation.

In lateral radiographs, the cardiac silhouette should span between 2.5 (deep-chested breeds) and 3.5 intercostal spaces. The angle between the trachea and spine varies by breed, but generally speaking, if the trachea runs parallel to the spine (dorsal displacement), cardiomegaly is present (Figs. 34 and 36). In the dorsoventral view, the cardiac silhouette occupies 60 to 65 % of the width of the thorax. A normal vertebral heart score (VHS) is between 8.5 and 10.5. This is a useful way to measure heart size. It is calculated by measuring the heart axes (long and short) on a lateral view, superimposing these lengths onto the spine starting at T4, and counting the vertebrae that fall within the range covered. A VHS over 12 in dogs with mitral insufficiency indicates a high risk of CHF.

Radiographs are useful to identify LA enlargement. Moderate to severe LA enlargement is detected on the lateral view by elevation of the carina and of the caudodorsal cardiac silhouette, and by the caudal border of the cardiac silhouette becoming straight instead of curving cranially (Fig. 34). The dorsoventral view shows a protrusion in the contour of the cardiac silhouette between two and three o'clock (clock face analogy) (Fig. 35). A wider space can be seen between the primary bronchi, with a double opacity between them.

In patients with left-sided CHF, the pulmonary vein may be thicker than the pulmonary arteries. Patients with right-sided CHF may have a dilated CaVC.

One of the main uses of thoracic radiographs in cardiac patients is to detect pulmonary oedema. The increase in extravascular fluid in the lungs appears as a diffuse increase in radiopacity of the caudodorsal lung fields (unstructured interstitial or alveolar pattern). An increase in perihilar radiopacity results from pulmonary oedema (Figs. 36 and 37) and pulmonary vein dilation near the LA. If the patient has severe dyspnoea, positioning for radiographs may be dangerous, so it is better to wait until the patient improves. Thoracic ultrasound is preferred in emergency cases for detecting oedema.

ELECTROCARDIOGRAPHY

The main use of electrocardiography (ECG) in dogs with CHF is identification of arrhythmias. The predominance of sympathetic tone means sinus tachycardia is more common than respiratory sinus arrhythmia in CHF patients.

Supraventricular and ventricular tachyarrhythmias are the most common rhythm disorders in dogs with CHF.

Myocardial lesions due to inflammation, ischaemia, or hypoxia can induce arrhythmogenic mechanisms like re-entry, abnormal automaticity, and after depolarisations that may lead to tachyarrhythmias.

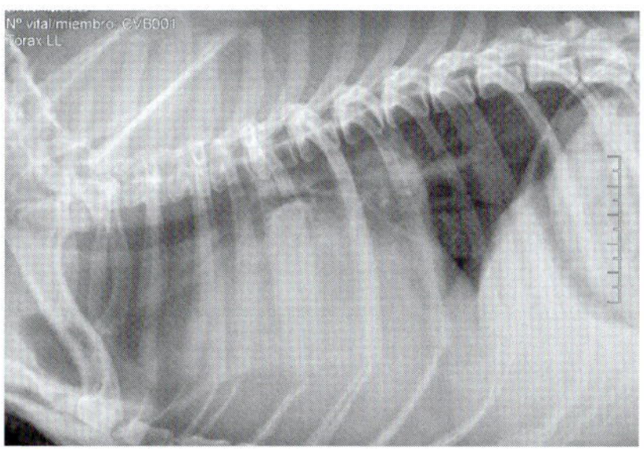

Figure 34. Lateral view. Severe generalised cardiomegaly with left atrial dilation. Patient with severe mitral insufficiency.

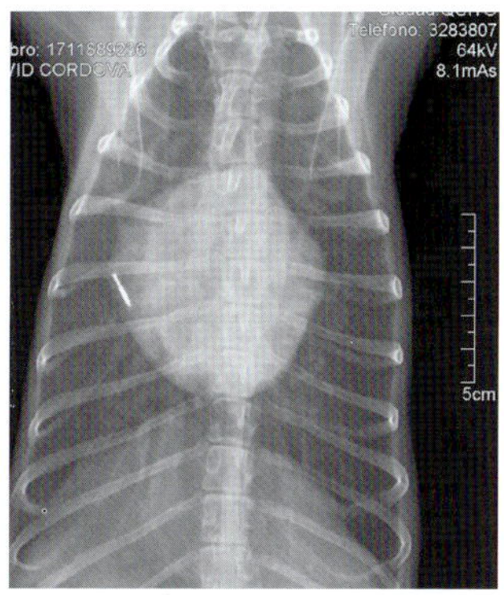

Figure 35. Lateral view. Left atrial dilation.

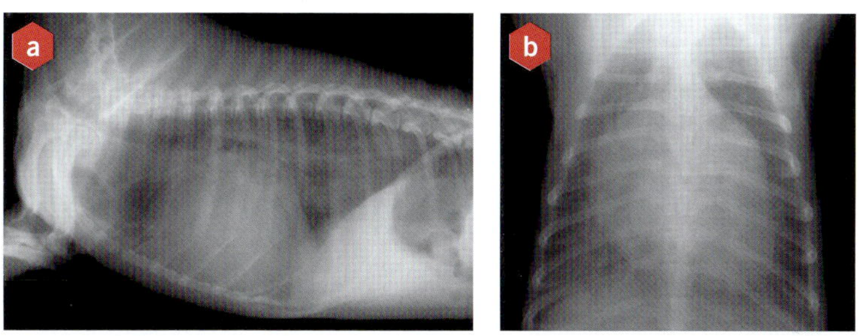

Figure 36. Lateral (a) and dorsoventral (b) views. Severe generalised cardiomegaly with signs of pulmonary oedema. Patient with mitral and tricuspid insufficiency.

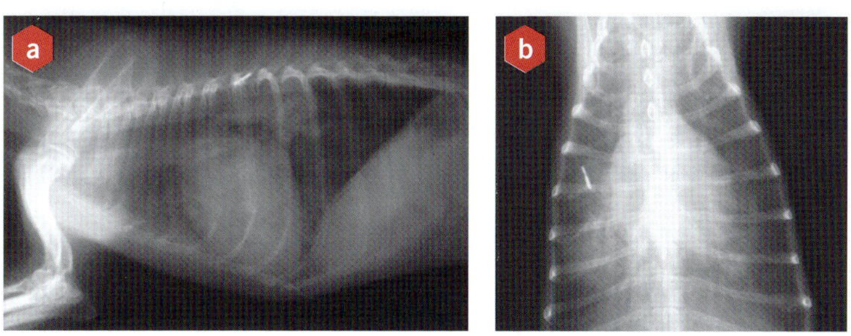

Figure 37. Lateral (a) and dorsoventral (b) views. Mild to moderate cardiomegaly with signs of pulmonary oedema. Patient with mitral insufficiency.

Supraventricular tachyarrhythmias

Supraventricular arrhythmias may present as single premature complexes (Fig. 38), as couplets, or possibly as tachycardia (sustained or not) (Fig. 39). Premature complexes are not usually associated with clinical signs, but high-frequency sustained tachycardia is often related to low cardiac output or congestive signs.

Atrial fibrillation is one of the most common tachyarrhythmias in dogs with severe atrial dilation. Loss of atrial contraction associated with increased frequency of ventricular depolarisation indicates haemodynamic and clinical worsening. Patients presenting with this arrhythmia tend to have CHF and ascites. This arrhythmia is characterised by a markedly irregular rhythm, a lack of P-waves, and, in some patients, F-waves (fine, irregular movements from baseline) (Figs. 40 and 41). QRS complexes tend to look supraventricular (narrow), but they can be wide in patients with LV hypertrophy or left bundle branch block. Heart rate tends to be very fast due to the increased sympathetic tone in patients with CHF.

The main therapeutic goal is to maintain a heart rate below 160 beats per minute (bpm). Conversion to sinus rhythm is possible with electric cardioversion or antiarrhythmics, but dogs with very enlarged LAs cannot sustain sinus rhythm over a longer period.

Ventricular arrhythmias

Ventricular arrhythmias are common in dogs with CHF and are a clinical feature of dogs with cardiomyopathy. They may appear as single premature complexes (Figs. 41 and 42), couplets, and sustained or nonsustained tachycardia. These may be wide, abnormal premature complexes with T waves opposite in polarity to the QRS complex and without associated P waves.

The severity of ventricular arrhythmias is based on the number of premature complexes, the frequency of depolarisation of the ectopic focus (Fig. 43), the presence of polymorphic complexes, the presence of rapid sustained tachycardia (Fig. 44) and the R-on-T phenomenon. Severe or malignant arrhythmias can cause haemodynamic instability and signs of low cardiac output; since they increase the risk of sudden death, they should be treated. Congestive heart failure treatment aims to mitigate the severity of ventricular arrhythmias.

While ECG is not a sensitive indicator of cardiac remodelling, ECG signs suggestive of it may appear in some patients. Left ventricular dilation and hypertrophy may increase the amplitude (Fig. 45) or duration of the R wave (above 2.5-3 mV or longer than 0.06 s). Left atrial dilation may widen the P wave (to longer than 0.04 s) and create a notch in it (P-mitrale). Right ventricular dilation and hypertrophy may cause right axis deviation, characterised by deep S waves in leads I, II, III and aVF.

Congestive heart failure patients may present with myocardial ischaemia or hypoxia that manifests as ST depression or elevation. Ischaemic areas may produce arrhythmogenic foci.

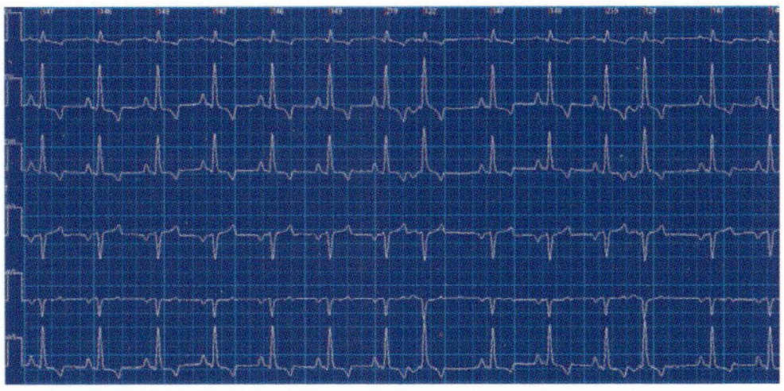

Figure 38. Beats 8 and 12 are supraventricular premature complexes. Patient with CHF secondary to mitral insufficiency.

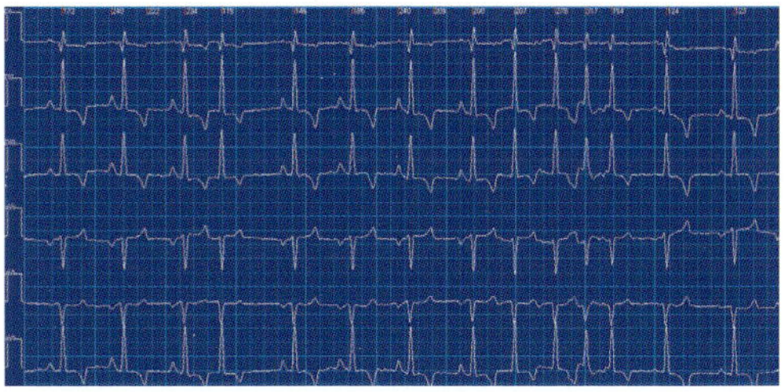

Figure 39. Beat 4 is a supraventricular premature complex. Beat 9 is the start of nonsustained supraventricular tachycardia. Patient with CHF secondary to mitral insufficiency.

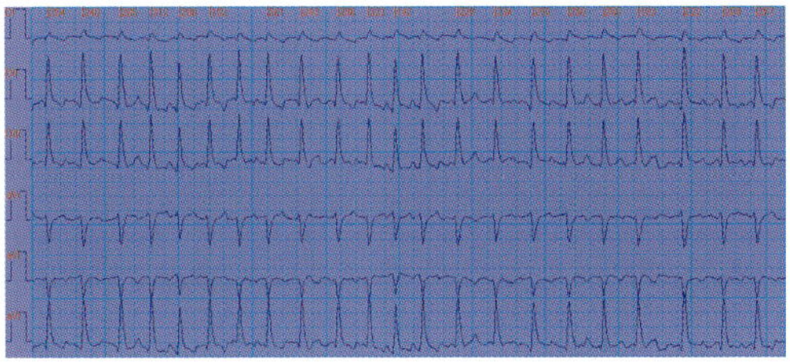

Figure 40. Atrial fibrillation with a rate of 280 bpm.

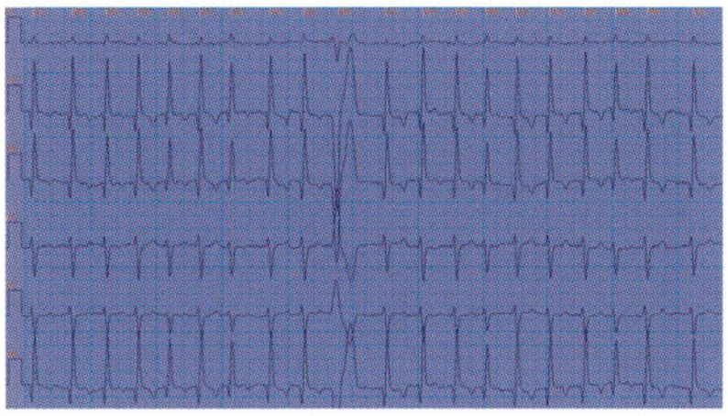

Figure 41. Atrial fibrillation at 240 bpm and a ventricular premature complex. Dog with CHF secondary to mitral insufficiency.

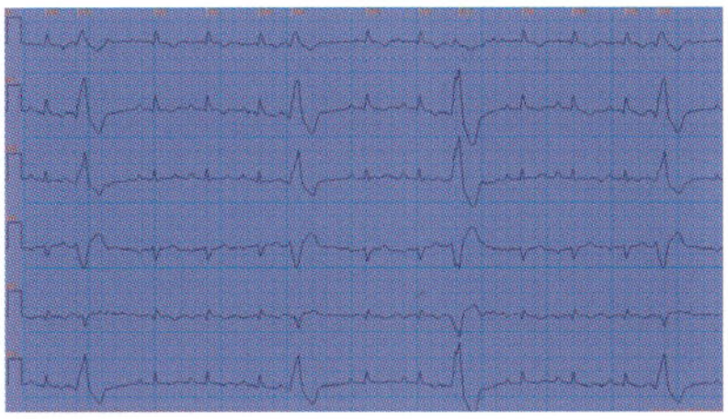

Figure 42. Premature ventricular complexes with positive polarity (leads I, II, III, aVf) in a Boxer with arrhythmogenic right ventricular cardiomyopathy.

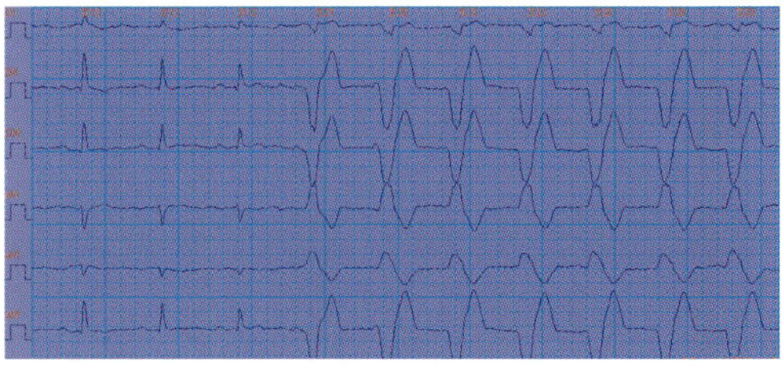

Figure 43. Start of slow sustained ventricular tachycardia with an ectopic depolarisation rate of 120–130 bpm. Patient with congestive heart failure and digoxin toxicity.

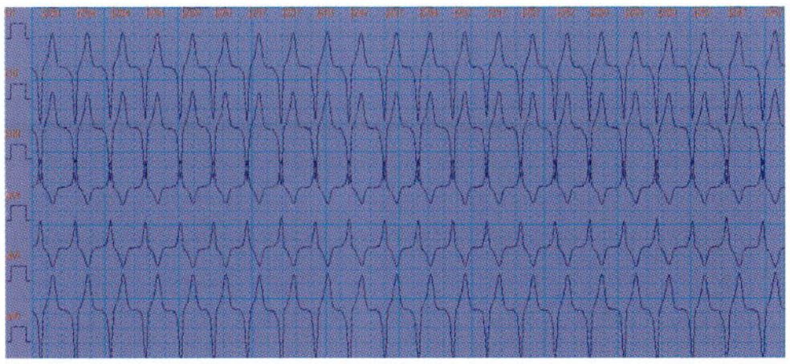

Figure 44. Sustained ventricular tachycardia at 250 bpm. Severe arrhythmia requiring aggressive treatment. Patient with cardiomyopathy.

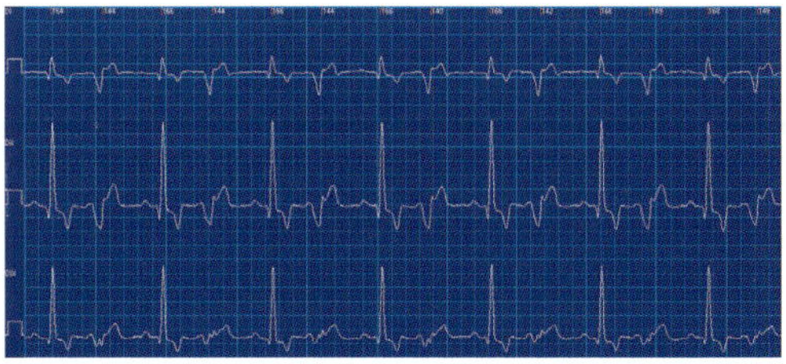

Figure 45. Ventricular bigeminy in a dog with CHF secondary to a patent ductus arteriosus. R-wave amplitude is very high (6 mV).

TREATMENT PRINCIPLES

Rational treatment is based on the pathophysiological principles of the disease, the available medical evidence, and the doctor's clinical experience.

> The owner should be informed of the importance of treatment and the consequences of noncompliance.

The owner should be aware that this treatment is lifelong, not curative, with the goal of improving the quality of life and the expected survival. The owner must also know the potential risks of treatment and inform the veterinary surgeon of any clinical changes seen in the patient.

Both emergency and long-term treatments can be considered. Patients requiring emergency care may fall into two categories: those with a previous diagnosis of and possible treatment for heart disease who have decompensated, and patients without a prior heart disease diagnosis.

The ACVIM functional classification system may assist clinicians in therapeutic decision-making.

EMERGENCY TREATMENT

Oxygen therapy

Dyspnoeic patients must be managed carefully in the emergency department, especially during diagnostic tests. Supplemental oxygen should be provided before determining the cause of dyspnoea and giving specific treatment; minimise stress in handling the patient. Severe pulmonary oedema can lead to severe hypoxaemia, along with decreases in oxygen intake and cellular energy production. Forced oxygen (e.g. mask oxygen therapy in an anxious, resistant patient) increases anxiety and muscular effort, at which point the benefits of oxygen therapy are outweighed by increased energy demand and consumption.

Initial supplementation may consist of humidified nasal flow-by oxygen. Small and medium dogs can then be placed in an oxygen chamber, while large dogs should be placed on oxygen with a nasal cannula. The humidified oxygen flow should be as follows:

- Nasal cannula: between 50 and 100 ml/kg/min.
- Chamber: between 6 and 10 l/min. Verify that the chamber does not become dangerously hot (ideal temperature: 18.5–22°C).

Ventilatory support

While mild to moderate pulmonary oedema is generally responsive to treatment, patients with severe dyspnoea may die of respiratory failure. Severe hypoxaemia can cause respiratory muscle fatigue, making mechanical ventilation unsustainable. The high risk of cardiopulmonary arrest in this situation necessitates aggressive therapy including life support measures such as mechanical ventilation, with the goal of easing the toll on the respiratory muscles and cardiovascular system. Mechanical ventilation keeps airways patent and protected, allowing fluid drainage from the airways and recruitment of unstable lung areas, thus enhancing alveolar ventilation.

Endotracheal intubation should be performed as quickly as possible without impacting haemodynamics; thus, a rapid intubation protocol is advised. This protocol involves intravenous (IV) administration of a combination of midazolam, fentanyl, and a nondepolarising neuromuscular blocker such as rocuronium or vecuronium.

Support respiration with the following measures:

- Limit the tidal volume (below 10 ml/kg, ideally 6–8 ml/kg) or the peak inspiratory pressure (no more than 25–30 cmH_2O, generally around 20 cmH_2O).
- Positive end expiratory pressure (PEEP) should be no less than 5–8 cmH_2O.
- The inspiratory pressure should be between 15 and 20 cmH_2O.
- The respiratory rate should be between 8 and 15 bpm, to a maximum of 20 bpm.
- Inspiratory time should not exceed 1–1.2 seconds.
- The fraction of inspired oxygen can go as high as 50 %.

The strategic goal is to recruit unstable alveoli with minimal risk of inducing lung damage (from hyperinflation and collapse and reopening of alveoli).

Ventilatory support should be provided for several hours to one day, until the medication achieves fluid drainage from the airways and decreases pulmonary oedema. The patient may then be placed in an oxygen chamber.

Drainage of effusions

Thoracocentesis is necessary for dyspnoeic patients with massive pleural effusion. The decrease in fluid in the pleural cavity often leads to significant clinical improvement. Abdominocentesis can improve ventilation and greatly help patients with severe ascites.

Anxiety control

Anxiety can be controlled with acepromazine at a dose of 0.01–0.03 mg/kg. Acepromazine decreases anxiety, improving patient welfare without depressing respiration. This drug, an α-adrenergic antagonist, has a vasodilating effect and decreases cardiac afterload, thus alleviating systolic wall stress. However, it can also cause hypotension. To prevent hypotension, first confirm that patients are normotensive and give the minimum effective dose.

Furosemide

In emergencies, IV furosemide is preferred; if IV is considered unsafe, intramuscular administration is also permissible, but it will act more slowly.

> The clinical goals of furosemide are reached when diuresis increases, respiratory rate decreases, and the breathing pattern improves.

Intravenous furosemide takes effect after 5 minutes and peaks at 30 minutes. However, the effect ends after approximately 2–3 hours, so patients who do not improve should receive repeat IV doses every 1–2 hours until the respiratory rate decreases. Once the patient improves, administer furosemide every 8 hours.

The canine dose is 1–4 mg/kg, based on severity and initial bolus response (higher doses are reserved for more severely ill patients). A constant rate infusion (CRI) of 1 mg/kg/h is an option in patients with severe signs who do not respond adequately to the initial bolus. A CRI may be more effective than a bolus for achieving diuresis and sodium and calcium excretion (with minimal potassium excretion).

Dobutamine

Dobutamine is a synthetic β-agonist catecholamine used as a positive inotrope. It can be given to patients with signs of low cardiac output, refractory CHF, and/or myocardial insufficiency.

It is given as a 5–10 µg/kg/min CRI (maximum 20 µg/kg/min). Doses are initially low and increased every 15–30 minutes until tissue perfusion improves.

It is important to consider the risks of vasodilation and hypotension due to its β2-adrenergic activity, as well as the risks of tachycardia and arrhythmogenesis at higher doses.

Sodium nitroprusside

Nitroprusside is an arterial and venous vasodilator that decreases cardiac preload and afterload. The decrease in venous pressure impedes the development of pulmonary oedema, and the decrease in systemic vascular resistance favours anterograde flow and lowers the mitral regurgitant fraction.

This drug is recommended in patients with severe pulmonary oedema who do not respond to initial treatment.

It is given as a 0.5–10 µg/kg/min CRI. The initial dose is low and is increased until the systemic blood pressure decreases by approximately 10 %. Sodium nitroprusside is given for up to 48 hours. The primary risk is hypotension, so blood pressure should be closely monitored.

Other potentially beneficial vasodilators include nitroglycerin gel, hydralazine, and amlodipine.

Initial therapy for severe CHF can be rewarding if diagnosis is rapid and treatment is goal-oriented.

LONG-TERM TREATMENT

Diuretics

Furosemide

Diuretics are the most effective drugs for controlling pulmonary oedema, ascites, and CHF-induced pleural effusion. They act by promoting diuresis to reduce blood volume, thereby mitigating ventricular filling pressures and congestion. Furosemide has been the most commonly used veterinary diuretic for decades, and it remains a pillar of CHF drug treatment in dogs. It acts on the thick ascending limb of the loop of Henle by impeding the Na-K-2Cl cotransporter and blocking sodium, chloride, and water reabsorption; at the same time, it promotes potassium, hydrogen, calcium, and magnesium ion excretion. Other potential benefits for patients with CHF include venous dilation, bronchodilation, improved lymphatic flow through the thoracic duct, and increased renal blood flow.

Long-term furosemide is given orally at the minimum dose that keeps the patient clinically stable, with a normal respiratory rate and pattern and no evidence of effusion. Bioavailability is up to 50 %. It begins to act within one hour of administration and works for up to six hours. Doses are quite variable, ranging from 1 mg/kg every 48 hours to 4 mg/kg every 8 hours (even higher in certain cases). Once the acute pulmonary oedema is controlled, give furosemide 2 mg/kg two to three times daily; recheck renal function and electrolyte levels and verify the absence of oedema every 5–7 days.

The owner should monitor the patient's resting or sleeping respiratory rate to assist in determining the minimum effective dose. In patients without oedema, this respiratory rate should be below 35 bpm (ideally below 30 bpm). If the respiratory rate remains normal and pulmonary oedema does not occur, the dose can be tapered at each recheck until the veterinary surgeon determines that a further dose reduction risks a recurrence of oedema or effusions. In some cases, the dose must be increased to treat recurrent clinical signs (e.g. due to disease progression over time).

In order to exert its effects, furosemide must reach its site of action; however, decreased cardiac output and intense vasoconstriction in CHF patients can often lower renal blood flow and thereby reduce the amount of free drug in the renal tubular lumen. Because furosemide is 90 to 95 % plasma protein-bound, hypoalbuminaemia means an initially high free drug concentration in the tubular lumen. However, the amount of drug in the vascular space decreases rapidly, which reduces the tubular drug concentration and, hence, the degree of diuresis. In such cases, patients require high doses to significantly enhance diuresis.

The main secondary effects are pre-renal azotaemia, hyponatraemia, hypokalaemia, hypochloraemia, metabolic alkalosis, and increased renin secretion, along with the sequelae of these effects. Mild to moderate increases in urea are also common in patients receiving furosemide. However, as long as creatinine remains within normal limits, patients appear unaffected.

Pre-renal azotaemia can also result from severe dehydration and decreased renal perfusion due to cardiac disease. Renal hypoperfusion can lead to ischaemic renal injury.

If azotaemia occurs with appetite loss and vomiting, decrease the dose of furosemide or suspend treatment with furosemide and angiotensin-converting enzyme inhibitors (ACEIs); rehydrate with a 50:50 IV combination of 5 % dextrose and lactated Ringer's solution, supplemented with potassium chloride (a maintenance fluid volume should suffice). In these cases, limit fluid administration to minimise pulmonary oedema. If the patient is eating, dehydration and electrolyte imbalances are less significant complications.

Spironolactone

Spironolactone is a selective competitive antagonist of the aldosterone receptor and is thus considered a potassium-sparing diuretic. Aldosterone is closely linked to CHF progression: it increases blood volume through sodium and water reabsorption in the distal tubule, promotes myocardial and perivascular fibrosis, and alters endothelial function.

It is recommended in addition to ACEIs and furosemide for these reasons:

- Although ACEIs can decrease aldosterone concentration initially, aldosterone levels soon rise again. This phenomenon is known as aldosterone escape.
- Furosemide treatment is also known to increase aldosterone concentration.

Spironolactone's diuretic effect is insignificant, but it potentiates furosemide's action. One clinical study showed that adding spironolactone to conventional treatment (ACEIs, furosemide, and digoxin) in dogs with moderate to severe mitral insufficiency reduces the risks of death from cardiac causes and of CHF exacerbation. It should be used in long-term treatment of stage C mitral insufficiency patients along with conventional treatment (although consensus does not exist on this point), as well as refractory stage D patients (highly recommended). The dose is 0.25–2 mg/kg every 12–24 hours.

Angiotensin-converting enzyme inhibitors

Angiotensin-converting enzyme inhibitors (e.g. enalapril) reduce plasma concentrations of angiotensin II (by arteriolar and venous vasodilation) and decrease sodium and water retention by decreasing release of aldosterone.

Initial studies of enalapril showed good tolerance and therapeutic benefits for dogs with CHF. Addition of this drug to therapy with diuretics and digoxin improved the survival and quality of life of dogs with mitral insufficiency and dilated cardiomyopathy, offering clinical and haemodynamic benefits including decreased pulmonary capillary pressure compared with patients who received only diuretics.

Benazepril also improved patient survival and quality of life compared with placebo. The ability of enalapril to delay the onset of CHF in dogs with moderate to severe mitral insufficiency has also been studied; minimal to no benefit was observed.

Angiotensin-converting enzyme inhibitors should be given to patients with cardiac remodelling and no clinical signs of insufficiency, because chamber dilation indicates strong RAAS activation and blocking RAAS is known to slow the progression of the disease. Nonetheless, significant clinical benefits have not been demonstrated. One clinical study (the QUEST study) compared the survival time of dogs with CHF due to mitral regurgitation when given benazepril or pimobendan combined with conventional treatment. Survival was greater in the pimobendan group than in the benazepril group, but the quality of life was similar in both.

The ACVIM *Guidelines for the Diagnosis and Treatment of Canine Chronic Valvular Heart Disease* in dogs recommend the use of ACEIs for long-term treatment of dogs in stage C but not for treating acute pulmonary oedema in stage C patients. Administration of an ACEI together with furosemide reduces pulmonary capillary pressure more than treatment with furosemide alone. Stage B2 patients with marked LA dilation may benefit from treatment with an ACEI, since these drugs can moderately delay the onset of CHF; however, no consensus exists on their use in this situation.

Enalapril maleate is given orally and has a bioavailability of 60 %. Its peak plasma concentration occurs 3 to 4 hours after administration, and its effects last approximately 12 hours, with primarily renal elimination. The recommended dose is 0.5 mg/kg every 12 hours. Due to the risk of a decreased glomerular filtration rate and electrolyte alterations (primarily when combined with furosemide), urea, creatinine, and electrolyte levels must be monitored approximately one week after the start of treatment.

Pimobendan

Pimobendan is a positive inotrope and a vasodilator (inodilator). It acts by inhibiting phosphodiesterase III and sensitising contractile proteins to calcium (increased affinity of troponin C for calcium). It has the following effects:

- Improves myocardial contractility and relaxation.
- Induces arterial and venous dilation in both the pulmonary and systemic vasculature.
- Slightly decreases blood pressure and increases heart rate at high doses, though these effects are subtle.
- Decreases pulmonary capillary pressure and the average heart rate in dogs with CHF, without increasing the incidence of ventricular or supraventricular arrhythmias.
- Decreases sympathetic tone and the concentration of proinflammatory cytokines.
- Myocardial oxygen consumption is lower with pimobendan than with dobutamine.

The QUEST study evaluated the survival of dogs with CHF from mitral regurgitation treated with pimobendan or benazepril. In patients who received pimobendan, survival was greater, the heart shrank more, and fluid retention was lower. In that study, the quality of life was similar across both groups. Long-term pimobendan treatment is now recommended for patients with stage C mitral insufficiency.

The EPIC study showed that administering pimobendan to dogs with preclinical (stage B2) mitral insufficiency considerably delayed the onset of clinical signs of CHF. Thus, prompt pimobendan treatment is recommended for dogs with stage B2 mitral insufficiency.

The PROTECT study found that pimobendan delays the onset of CHF signs and decreases sudden death in Dobermans with occult dilated cardiomyopathy (preclinical), improving their survival. This study also demonstrated a reduction in the heart size without exacerbation of ventricular arrhythmias.

Thus, the experimental data support the use of pimobendan in emergency patients with acute pulmonary oedema.

The recommended dose is 0.2–0.3 mg/kg every 12 hours. The bioavailability is approximately 60 %, and plasma levels peak one hour after administration.

> The bioavailability of pimobendan decreases when it is given with food, so it should be given one hour before a meal.

Recommendations for pimobendan use

- QUEST study: Long-term treatment of patients with stage C mitral insufficiency.
- EPIC study: Early treatment of dogs with stage B2 mitral insufficiency.
- PROTECT study: Treatment of Dobermans with occult dilated cardiomyopathy.

Digoxin

Digoxin is an inhibitor of the Na-K-ATPase pump that can normalise baroreceptor function. It is a mild positive inotrope that mitigates autonomic dysfunction (increases vagal activity and lessens sympathetic tone) and slows the heart rate.

Its current clinical indication is controlling the heart rate in certain patients with atrial fibrillation, although diltiazem or amiodarone is usually necessary for control. It is also used for moderate inotropic support of dogs with myocardial insufficiency who present with advanced (stage C or D) CHF; however, pimobendan has replaced digoxin as the primary positive inotrope.

The maintenance dose in dogs below 20 kg is 0.005–0.011 mg/kg every 12 hours, and in dogs over 20 kg it is 0.22 mg/m^2 every 12 hours.

To check serum drug levels, take a sample between days 4 and 7, 8–12 hours after dosing. The therapeutic range is 0.8–2.0 ng/ml.

Several factors and drugs interact with digoxin to alter its metabolism, absorption, excretion, and volume of distribution. Dose reduction should be considered in patients with kidney disease, hypothyroidism, hypoalbuminaemia, loss of muscle mass, and ascites. Hypokalaemia increases myocardial digoxin concentration and predisposes patients to cardiotoxicity. Drugs that alter its pharmacokinetics include verapamil, amiodarone, spironolactone, phenobarbital, aspirin, furosemide, and hydrochlorothiazide, and low-sodium diets also affect its pharmacokinetics. Beta blockers and calcium channel blockers enhance its vagal effects.

The initial signs of toxicity are anorexia, depression, vomiting, and diarrhoea. Cardiac toxicity may manifest as sinus bradycardia, AV block of varying grades, ventricular tachycardia or bigeminy, and supraventricular arrhythmias.

Sildenafil

The drug of choice for pulmonary hypertension is sildenafil citrate. It is a selective pulmonary vasodilator that acts by inhibiting phosphodiesterase V, the enzyme responsible for inactivating the GMPc produced by the nitric oxide pathway; nitric oxide is both a vasodilator and an inhibitor of cellular proliferation. In pulmonary hypertension, GMPc activity is decreased in proportion to an increase in phosphodiesterase V, which is found in high concentrations in the pulmonary endothelium. Sildenafil increases GMPc, leading to haemodynamic and clinical improvement. It has been shown to mitigate the severity of pulmonary hypertension and improve quality of life and survival. The dose is 1–3 mg/kg every 8–12 hours.

Antiarrhythmics

The most common arrhythmias associated with CHF are supraventricular tachyarrhythmias and ventricular arrhythmias. Treatment is necessary if these cause clinical or haemodynamic deterioration or if they pose a risk of sudden death. Severe supraventricular tachycardias can be treated with digoxin, diltiazem, or amiodarone. The primary goal of treating atrial fibrillation is to keep the heart rate below 160 bpm. Using cardioversion to recover a sinus rhythm does not ensure a better clinical course than simply controlling the rate does. When treatment is initiated with digoxin, additional drugs such as diltiazem or amiodarone may be necessary for adequate rate control.

Severe ventricular arrhythmias associated with advanced heart disease must be treated. Treatment options include atenolol with mexiletine and class III antiarrhythmics such as sotalol or amiodarone. Amiodarone is given at a starting dose of 10 mg/kg every 12 hours and reduced to 5 mg/kg every 12 hours after 1–2 weeks.

Beta blockers

To protect the myocardium from the damaging effects of excessive sympathetic tone, β-adrenergic blockers such as atenolol and β- and α-adrenergic blockers such as carvedilol can be administered, mainly in dogs with dilated cardiomyopathy.

These are also used to control the heart rate in atrial fibrillation. Long-term administration has been shown to protect the myocardium and improve ventricular systolic function in humans, but the same effects have not been seen in dogs.

These drugs are not indicated in CHF patients. It they are used in patients with subclinical disease, pimobendan should be given simultaneously to prevent their potential negative inotropic effects.

DIETARY CONSIDERATIONS

A moderate decrease in salt intake is recommended in patients with stage C and D CHF. Limiting salt consumption can moderate the increase in plasma volume. The sodium content of the selected diet should be 10 to 40 mg/kg of dry food.

Ensure an adequate caloric intake (60 kcal/kg body weight) and a sufficient protein intake to prevent cardiac cachexia. In case of inappetence or anorexia, determine the cause (azotaemia, drug toxicity, etc.) and make the necessary changes to aid the patient.

LONG-TERM DRUG TREATMENT

Stage of CHF		Recommended	Optional
Stage A		Treatment is not recommended.	-
Stage B	B1	Treatment is not recommended.	-
	B2	Pimobendan, ACEIs.	Salt restriction.
Stage C		Furosemide, pimobendan, ACEIs. Salt restriction.	Spironolactone, digoxin, beta blockers, diltiazem, amiodarone, cough suppressants, bronchodilators.
Stage D		Furosemide, pimobendan, ACEIs, spironolactone. Salt restriction.	Digoxin, hydrochlorothiazide, sildenafil, beta blockers, diltiazem, amiodarone, cough suppressants, bronchodilators.

REFERENCES

Abbott LM, Kovacic J. The pharmacologic spectrum of furosemide. *Journal of Veterinary Emergency and Critical Care*. 2008; 26–39.

Adin D, Atkins C, Papich M et al. Furosemide continuous rate infusion diluted with 5% dextrose in water or hypertonic saline in normal adult dogs: a pilot study. *Journal of Veterinary Cardiology*. 2017; 44–56.

Atkins CE, Keene BW, Brown WA et al. Results of the veterinary enalapril trial to prove reduction in onset of heart failure in dogs chronically treated with enalapril alone for compensated, naturally occurring mitral valve insufficiency (Vetproof). *Journal of the American Veterinary Medical Association*. 2007; 1061–1069.

Atkins C, Bonagura J, Ettinger S et al. Guidelines for the diagnosis an treatment of canine chronic valvular herat disease. *Journal of Veterinary Internal Medicine*. 2009; 1–9.

Bach JF, Rozanski EA, MacGregor J et al. Retrospective Evaluation of Sildenafil Citrate as a Therapy for Pulmonary Hypertension in Dogs. *Journal of Veterinary Internal Medicine*. 2006; 1132–1135.

Barr F and Gaschen L. *Manual of Canine and Feline Ultrasonography*. UK: BSAVA. 2012.

Bernay F, Bland J, Haggstrom J et al. Efficacy of spironolactone on survival in dogs with naturally occurring mitral regurgitation caused by myxomatous mitral valve disease. *Journal of Veterinary Internal Medicine*. 2010; 331–341.

Boon JA. *Veterinary Echocardiography*. UK: Wiley-Blackwell. 2011.

Borgarelli M, Crosara S, Lamb K et al. Survival characteristics and prognostic variables of dogs with preclinical chronic degenerative mitral valve disease attributable to myxomatous degeneration. *Journal of Veterinary Internal Medicine*. 2012; 69–75.

Borgarelli M, Abbott J, Braz-Ruivo L et al. Prevalence and prognostic importance of pulmonary hypertension in dogs with myxomatous mitral valve disease. *Journal of Veterinary Internal Medicine*. 2015; 569–574.

Boswood A, Haggstrom J, Gordon S et al. Effect of pimobendan in dogs with preclinical myxomatous mitral valve disease and cardiomegaly: the EPIC study-A randomized clinical trial. *Journal of Veterinary Internal Medicine*. 2016; 1765–1779.

Bright J and zum Brunnen J. Chronicity of atrial fibrillation affects duration of sinus rhythm after transthoracic cardioversion of dogs with naturally occurring atrial fibrillation. *Journal of Veterinary Internal Medicine*. 2008; 114–119.

Ettinger S, Benitz A, Ericsson G et al. Effects of enalapril maleate on survival of dogs with naturally acquired heart failure. The long-term investigation of veterinary enalapril (live) study group. *Journal of the American Veterinary Medical Asociation*. 1998; 1573–1577.

Fuentes VL. Use of pimobendan in the management of heart failure. *Veterinary Clinics Small Animal Practice*. 2004; 1145–1155.

Gelzer A and Kraus M. Management of atrial fibrillation. *Veterinary Clinics Small Animal Practice*. 2004; 1127–1144.

Goutal CM, Keir I, Kenney S et al. Evaluation of acute congestive heart failure in dogs and cats: 145 cases (2007-2008). *Journal of Veterinary Emergency and Critical Care*. 2010; 330–337.

Haggstrom J, Boswood A, O'Grady M et al. Effect of pimobendan or benazepril hydrochloride on survival times in dogs with congestive heart failture caused by naturally occurring myxomatous mitral valve disease: the QUEST study. *Journal of Veterinary Internal Medicine*. 2008; 1124–1135.

Haggstrom J, Hoglund K and Borgarelli M. An update on treatment and prognostic indicators in canine myxomatous mitral valve disease. *Journal of Small Animal Practice*. 2009; 25–33.

Haggstrom J, Boswood A, O'Grady M et al. Longitudinal analysis of quality of life, clinical, radiographic, echocardiographic, and laboratory variables in dogs with myxomatous mitral valve disease receiving pimobendan or benazepril: the QUEST study. *Journal of Veterinary Internal Medicine*. 2013; 1441–1451.

Hezzell M, Boswood A, Chang Y-M et al. The combined prognostic potential of serum high-sensitivity cardiac troponin I and N-terminal pro-B-type natriuretic peptide concentrations in dogs with degenerative mitral valve disease. *Journal of Veterinary Internal Medicine*. 2012; 302–311.

Hezzell MJ, Boswood A, Lotter N et al. The effects of storage conditions on measurements of canine N-terminal pro-B-type natriuretic peptide. *Journal of Veterinary Cardiology*. 2015; 34–41.

Hogan D. The effect of benazepril on survival times and clinical sings of dogs with congestive heart failture: Results of a multicenter, prospective, randomized, double-blinded, placebo-controlled, long-term clinical trial. *Journal of Veterinary Cardiology*. 1999; 7–18.

Kellihah HB, Stepien RL. Pulmonary hypertension in canine degenerative mitral valve disease. *Journal of Veterinary Cardiology*. 2012; 149–164.

Kittleson MD, Kienle RD. *Medicina cardiovascular de pequeños animales*. Barcelona-Spain: Multimédica. 2000.

Kvart C, Haggstrom J, Pedersen HD et al. Efficacy of enalapril for prevention of congestive heart failure in dogs with myxomatous valve disease and asymptomatic mitral regurgitation (Svep). *Journal of Veterinary Internal Medicine*. 2002; 80–88.

Lake-Bakaar GA, Singh MK, Kass PH et al. Effect of pimobendan on the incidence of arrhythmias in small breed dogs with myxomatous mitral valve degeneration. *Journal of Veterinary Cardiology.* 2015; 120–128.

Mattoon JS, Nyland TG. *Diagnóstico ecográfico en pequeños animales.* Barcelona-Spain: Gráfica IN Multimédica, S.A. 2016.

Mizuno M, Yamano S, Chimura S et al. Efficay of pimobendan on survival and reoccurrence of pulmonary edema in canine congestive heart failure. *The Journal of Veterinary Medical Science.* 2017; 29–34.

O'Grady M, O'Sullivan M. Dilated cardiomyopathy: an update. *Veterinary Clinics Small Animal Practice.* 2004; 1187–1207.

Oyama M. Neurohormonal activation in canine degenerative mitral valve disease: implications on pathophysiology and treatment. *Journal of Small Animal Practice.* 2009; 3–11.

Oyama MA, Boswood A, Connolly DJ et al. Clinical usefulness of an assay of measurement of circulating N-terminal pro-B-type natriuretic peptide concentration in dogs and cats with heart disease. *Journal of the American Veterinary Medical Association.* 2013; 71–82.

Porciello F, Rishniw M, Ljungvall I et al. Sleeping and resting respiratory rates in dogs and cats with medically-controlled left-sided congestive heart failure. *The Veterinary Journal.* 2016; 164–168.

Pouchelon J-L, Jamet N, Gouni V et al. Effect of benazepril on survival and cardiac events in dogs with asymtomatic mitral valve disease: a retrospective study of 141 cases. *Journal of Veterinary Internal Medicine.* 2008; 905–914.

Pouchelon J, Atkins C, Bussadori C et al. Cardiovascular-renal axis disorders in the domestic dog and cat: a veterinary consensus statement. *Journal of Small Animal Practice.* 2015; 537–552.

Sargent J, Muzzi R, Mukherjee R et al. Echocardiographic predictors of survival in dogs with myxomatous mitral valve disease. *Journal of Veterinary Cardiology.* 2015; 1–12.

Schober K, Hart T, Stern J et al. Detection of congestive heart failure in dogs by doppler echocardiography. *Journal of Veterinary Internal Medicine.* 2010; 1358–368.

Schwarz T, Johnson V. *Manual de diagnóstico por imagen del tórax en pequeños animales.* Barcelona-Spain: Ediciones S. 2013.

Sisson D. Neuroendocrine evaluation of cardiac disease. *Veterinary Clinics Small Animal Practice.* 2004; 1105–1126.

Smith FW, Tilley LP, Oyama MA et al. *Manual de cardiología canina y felina.* Barcelona-Spain: Elsevier. 2016.

Summerfield N, Boswood A, O'Grady M et al. Efficacy of pimobendan in the prevention of congestive heart failure or sudden death in doberman pinscher with preclinical dilated cardiomyopathy (the PROTECT Study). *Journal of Veterinary Internal Medicine.* 2012; 1337–1349.

Suzuki S, Fukushima R, Ishikawa T et al. The effect of pimobendan on left atrial pressure in dogs with mitral valve regurgitation. *Journal of Veterinary Internal Medicine.* 2011; 1328–33.

Vezzosi T, Mannucci T, Pistoresi A et al. Assessment of lung ultrasound B-lines in dogs with different stages of chronic valvular heart disease. *Journal of Veterinary Internal Medicine.* 2017; 700–704.

Wolf J, Gerlach N, Weber K et al. Lowered N-terminal pro-B-type natriuretic peptide levels in response to treatment predict survival in dogs with symptomatic mitral valve disease. *Journal of Veterinary Cardiology.* 2012; 399–408.

Woodfield JA, Bauer T, Rush JE et al. Acute and short-term hemodynamic, echocardiographic, and clinical effects of enalapril maleate in dogs with naturally acquired heart failure: results of the invasive multicenter prospective veterinary evaluation of enalapril study (Improve). *Journal of Veterinary Internal Medicine.* 1995; 234–242.

Woodfield J, Bauer T, Ettinger S et al. Controlled clinical evaluation of enalapril in dogs with heart failure: results of the cooperative veterinary enalapril (Cove) study group. *Journal of Veterinary Internal Medicine.* 1995; 243–252.